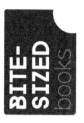

Bite-Sized Books

Eden is Burning – What Next for the NHS?

Peter McLardy-Smith

Cover by

Dean Stockton

Published by Bite-Sized Books Ltd 2022

GH00468155

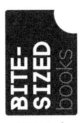

Bite-Sized Books Ltd 8th Floor, 20 St. Andrews Street, London EC4A 3AY, UK

Registered in the UK. Company Registration No: 9395379

ISBN: 9798412593944

For

My Wife and Children

Acknowledgments

Several of the thoughts, observations and suggestions recorded in this book have evolved over many years of conversations with a lot of friends and colleagues, but I should mention a few with whom I have spent the most time discussing the difficulties of health care delivery. These include Professor Nick Athanasou, Sr. Vicky Flanagan, Professor Max Gibbons, Dr. Simon Ostlere and Dr. David Pigott.

Others have helped with the Manuscript. Without the technical expertise and encouragement of Barbara Marks it would probably never have been completed.

The studies discussed in chapter 2 were brought to my attention in a presentation by Professor Kjell Haug of the University of Bergen, at a meeting organized by a friend, Professor Lars Engeseter. They kindly provided access to the data.

And for sage advice on style and content I must thank, among others, Dr. Viscountess Bearsted, Nick Beringer, Johnny Carmichael, Catherine Grubb, Dr. Claire Harries, Andrew Merton and Charlotte Weychan.

Finally, with the process of publication, I am indebted to Professor Sir Muir Gray, Christopher Gray of The Oxford Times and Julian Costley and Paul Davies of Bite-Sized Books.

Contents

Foreword

> "Gentlemen, he said
> I don't need your organization, I've shined your shoes
> I've moved your mountains and marked your cards
> But Eden is burning, either brace yourself for elimination
> Or your hearts must have the courage for the changing of
> the guards".
>
> This is the penultimate verse of a song by Bob Dylan called
> "Changing of the Guards", released on the album "Street-Legal" in June
> 1978.

There is debate about what was on Dylan's mind when he wrote it, but there is no way he could have been thinking about Health Care delivery for The United Kingdom in the 21st Century. Such is often the power of his imagery, however, that it can be applied to several situations. I believe that these would be the sentiments of virtually every employee of the NHS involved in direct patient contact towards those in the target obsessed and often clinically clueless management and administration systems.

Since its inception the NHS has survived on the goodwill and commitment of its clinical staff (by "clinical" I mean everyone involved directly in patient treatment, communication and comfort; from GP's and their receptionists in the community to consultants and cleaners in the hospitals).

But that goodwill is almost exhausted, morale is at rock-bottom and staff are leaving the NHS in droves, often reluctantly, for better paid and less stressful, though less rewarding, jobs.

The ongoing Coronavirus Pandemic of 2020 has made the public aware of the stressful nature of working in the health care "frontline", changing the previous attitude of indifference, or even petulant resentment, to one of gratitude. That may last, although I think it unlikely. Through 2021 the frustrations of waiting times have been heightened by the shift in clinical priorities consequent upon the pandemic dramas of the previous year. In any case, gratitude does not pay the rent. There are many parts of the country where people simply cannot afford to live working on a nurse or therapist's salary.

Inept politicians of all Parties vie with each other as to who will promise the most money to pour into the black hole which the NHS has now become. Yet there are people, from individuals to institutions and corporations, who make vast sums of money out of health care, almost invariably at the expense of the NHS. These financial injustices must be reversed.

If the NHS is to survive, all these financial problems and many cultural ones must be properly, sometimes radically, addressed, not just papered over as happens at present. The NHS has become like an evil charity, always in need of more money; but a tiny proportion of the money received actually benefits the community which it purports to serve.

I am not (and have no wish to be) an economist, sociologist or investigative journalist, but I have worked in the NHS for over 40 years and, in that time, I have seen many practices that are stupid, inefficient, venal or even dangerous. In this book I want to discuss some of those practices and suggest changes to them and to the whole structure and ethos of the NHS and its relationship with the Community. Perhaps Eden can still be saved from burning.

Oxford.

February 2022

Introduction

In the 1970's, on qualifying from Medical School we obtained preliminary registration with the GMC and did six months of hospital medicine as a pre-registration House Physician and six months of hospital surgery as a pre-registration House Surgeon. I really enjoyed my pre-registration jobs and, in that year, not surprisingly, I learnt more about being a doctor than in the previous three years as a clinical medical student. It also gave newly qualified doctors the chance to choose what particular field they wanted to go into. We were then able to get full registration with the General Medical Council and start looking for post-registration jobs which would lead to a formal specific training programme. Broadly speaking these would be in one of specialist medicine including psychiatry, specialist surgery including trauma management, the majority would be in general practice and there were other smaller specialisations such as radiology and clinical science. My own inclination was to go broadly into the field of hospital surgery and, by chance rather than planning, I found myself drawn to, and supported in, the field of orthopaedic surgery. I should say that throughout this period (which lasted from 1978 – 1987) I felt, with a few brief exceptions, very well taught and supported. It was a good training programme and by and large I think it produced thoughtful, skilful and committed practitioners.

It involved working very long hours and the pay was poor. In both my pre-registration jobs I did a rota of one in two, meaning that I was on-call every second night and the following day; whether I had been up all night or not, I was expected to provide a normal day's service. I lived in the hospital, where the accommodation was provided (I couldn't afford to live anywhere else but wouldn't have wanted to anyway) and I was well fed and well cared for by the domestic staff. I felt, and was, privileged and valued.

Since that time the training programmes have been changed on many occasions and in many ways. One of the biggest changes was the imposition of the European Working Time Directive which restricts the number of hours per week that anybody can work at any job. When your job is partly to provide a service, but mainly to gain experience, the less time per week you spend doing it, the longer it will take you to learn. I do not think that the trainees coming off the top of their programme today have anything like the experience behind them that we had forty years ago.

Junior doctors are also now quite well paid, but hospital accommodation has largely disappeared. This has changed the whole social ethos of hospital life, in my opinion not for the better. I am not really able to say whether training programmes now are better or worse than in the old days but, not surprisingly, my belief is that they were better forty years ago, both medically and socially.

My consultant appointment was to specialise in the field of hip and knee joint replacement surgery and revisions of those devices that had failed for whatever reason. It was what had been my greatest interest during training and I did this to the exclusion of any other form of clinical practice for a little over thirty years. I enjoyed it enormously and continued to feel privileged and, most of the time, valued.

Whatever the comparative merits of different training programmes I have no doubt that within the NHS the practice of surgery is performed, on the whole, with more thought and compassion and with greater technical skill today than it was when I first started. It is certainly better regulated and that is a good response to an increased public insight and awareness (in attempting to discuss treatment options with a patient the response of "you know best Doctor" is, thankfully, now extinct), but paradoxically the public's appreciation of the service provided for them is dramatically less than it was thirty years ago. This is partly due, I feel, to a progressive societal malaise in which any misfortune, however great or small, must be somebody else's fault, together with an increasing inability to distinguish between a privilege and a right. I do not think anybody involved in working within the health care systems would want obsequious gratitude (we are just trying to be of service) but some degree of appreciation, rather than endless criticism, can be quite good for morale. This has been shown recently by the change in the public's attitude to healthcare workers induced by the coronavirus pandemic, but I doubt if that change of attitude will last.

If I was to say that I was lucky enough to really enjoy my job, it is not to say that I did not also encounter a number of frustrations in the working environment and over the last ten to fifteen years I have been beset by an increasing feeling that the whole of the NHS is drifting into a firewall of catastrophe. It has, I believe, now reached the point where it is in real danger of complete collapse and my thoughts as to why this should be have evolved over a number of years, culminating in my decision to attempt to write this book.

Most of the ideas were conceived long before the start of 2020, when nobody had heard of covid 19. The events of the pandemic will have wide- and far-reaching consequences to every aspect of life, but initially its impact has been on health care delivery and obviously it would be inappropriate not to try and incorporate those effects with my thoughts in this book. In general, those events have strengthened my opinions and reinforced the reasons for my conclusions.

I have only ever worked (and lived) in the south of England so my experiences are based on that region. I acknowledge that there are some structural differences in the NHS in Scotland and Northern Ireland, but I have no insight into them. Despite that I have chosen to use the title UK throughout the book. The NHS is a UK wide organisation which was instituted at the same time throughout the UK. There will inevitably be some regional variations in such a large and widespread institution, but I believe that, where appropriate, I remark on this.

Similarly, I admit that my own field of experience and expertise is the comparatively narrow one of highly specialised surgical practice and thus most of the examples I will give to illustrate the points I wish to make will be drawn, whether real or anecdotal, from my own experience. My insight into other specialist fields within the NHS and beyond is limited, but it is not possible to work in any aspect of health care without interacting with a wide spectrum of other clinical fields and I feel justified in the conclusions I draw and the solutions I suggest.

I also acknowledge that it is easy to identify problems and not so easy to find feasible solutions, but I believe that the identification of the problem is the first essential step towards finding its solution. Many of the problems in the NHS have become endemic and are conveniently ignored.

This is by no means a scientific book. At best it could be regarded as a thoughtful insight and analysis of some of the problems within the NHS, with a few innovative suggestions for their solution. At worst it could be thought a list of bitter complaints about insoluble paradoxes.

There are certainly a number of paradoxes within my thinking and my ideas. I like paradoxes. A person who finds no paradoxes within their belief structures is, in my opinion, likely to be something of a monomaniac, with an obsessive belief that they know all there is to know about a topic, which leads to blinded bigotry.

Although not a scientific work I think it is important to define precisely what I mean by certain terms which I will use throughout the book.

By health care delivery I mean the provision of all aspects of health care for the sick, injured, or disabled from cradle to grave. This includes, apart from the obvious things of dealing with acute or chronic illness, the long-term provision of care for the disabled, provision of care for mental wellbeing, and social care including care homes for the elderly and disabled. Physical care from cradle to grave is not every aspect of a welfare state as that includes financial care, education, law and order etc.

By clinician I mean all staff involved in patient diagnosis and management in a clinical setting. Obviously, this includes doctors, but it also includes nurses and physiotherapists, occupational therapists, clinical psychologists, etc. Anybody who makes a clinical management decision or provides a therapeutic intervention.

Front line worker is a term derived from the attempts to manage the coronavirus pandemic and in this book, I use it to mean all staff who have a direct physical or verbal contact with patients and patient wellbeing. For example, I use this to include clerical staff, secretarial staff, hospital porters, hospital cleaners; anybody who, by doing their job well (whether it be performing an operation, pushing a bed, sweeping a floor or providing guidance and advice on the telephone), can improve the patient's experience of their management. For example, it includes ambulance crew, but not fire and rescue teams or police officers, although those two may also be essential services at the scene of an accident.

Finally, I am aware that in writing a book like this, the very nature of which involves criticism of the attitudes, behaviour and culture of several groups of people or individuals (although only politicians are specifically named) involved in health care delivery, I am in danger of appearing somewhat hubristic. I have never been a committed strategist or manager, either self-seeking or self-effacing. As a clinician I was not a "rogue doctor", in any sense of the term, but neither was I any better or worse than the vast majority of my clinical colleagues. Like most of us, even the most ardently "risk averse", I based my disease management decisions on my experience, knowledge and expertise. Like all of us there were a few times when those decisions resulted in, for whatever reason, bad or disappointing outcomes, but for most of us the intention was always to serve the best interests of the patient. The only times, infrequently, when I encountered something other than those best interests was when clinicians were tempted to take on something outside their level of experience or field of expertise, when there was no need to do so.

That is hubris, but we are all human.

Chapter 1

A Millennium of Health Care in Britain ending in the NHS

In the entire United Kingdom, there is probably no subject that can provoke such strong and disparate opinions, from such a large proportion of the population, as the National Health Service. Everyone has had some, direct or indirect, experience of it on which they base their varying judgements. These range from almost sycophantic appreciation – "The envy of the world" – to disenchanted derision – "A national disgrace - on the point of collapse".

There is much about The UK of which we should, but often forget to, be very proud but I do not think that "envy of the world" is a realistic aspiration for any aspect of any nation's public life. Certainly not the NHS, anyway, the world is too diverse for such uniformity of opinion.

On the other hand, unlike our public transport systems or the preponderance of people who regard the entire country as a giant rubbish bin, it is certainly not "a national disgrace".

Clearly the truth must lie somewhere within this wide spectrum from incredibly good to unbelievably bad, but which side is the pendulum of reality closest to. Perhaps more importantly, in which direction is it swinging. This book is an attempt to answer those two questions and my intention is to show that it is closest to the good side. The NHS remains one of those things of which the nation should be proud, but I also intend to show that the pendulum is swinging, fast, towards the bad side. We are in danger of losing the NHS. It could become the weed-clogged mud at the bottom of the stream of health care delivery; if that happens it will be because the clear and flowing stream has been commercialised into a stagnant pond.

George Santayana, a Spanish philosopher who lived from 1863 to 1952, observed that "a society that forgets its past has no future". History is always a good starting point.

Aneurin Bevan is universally and appropriately acknowledged as the founding force behind the National Health Service, but the concept was not a new one. The earliest care for the sick or disabled was most often provided by religious foundations, the oldest still in existence in England being St Bartholomew's Hospital founded in the Priory of St Bartholomew in London in 1123. The foundation of monastic orders, some of great wealth, with the responsibility of a "hospital" attached to them seems to have been one of the better practices introduced by the Normans after Williams successful invasion of 1066. The hospitals provided care (nursing) for the sick, but there was, of course, little in the way of meaningful therapeutic interventions; they often also cared for the destitute, the poor, the aged and infirm, the insane and the homeless.

Following Henry VIII's dissolution of the monasteries many of these hospitals were taken over by secular bodies, funded either by wealthy and noble patronage or by Municipal Authorities. For instance, St. Bartholomew's was re-founded on secular lines by Henry VIII in 1544 and a petition from the citizens of London lead, in1546, to the hospital being granted to the City of London and a board of governors being set up to administer it. The basic constitution and functions of the hospitals remained largely unchanged until the industrial revolution, although the theory and practice of medicine and surgery, together with its teaching and regulation was gradually evolving into something more comparable with that established by the time of the creation of the NHS.

The practice of some form of medical or surgical intervention, whether or not it was to the benefit of the species involved, is probably as old as evolution. But we need only go back as far as the beginning of the 16th century to see the emergence of physicians and surgeons in the way that we now understand them. The College of Physicians of London was established by Royal Charter of Henry VIII in 1518. One of its purposes was said to be – believe it or not – to curb malpractice and expose charlatans. After 500 years we still have some way to go! More realistically, certainly more usefully and a contribution to achieving the first two aspirations, it was empowered to licence qualified practitioners. Becoming a Licentiate probably did not involve a lot more than serving time as an apprentice with an established physician, but it was a start.

In 1923, by Act of Parliament, it was extended to cover all of England, becoming The Royal College of Physicians of England. There are also, although I will not go into their history, Royal Colleges of Physicians in Edinburgh, Ireland (Dublin) and (combined with Surgeons) Glasgow. One must be a Member, by examination, of one or more of these Royal Colleges to practice as a specialist physician in Ireland or the UK.

Before 1518 the barber surgeons had already been incorporated as Guilds of The City of London and, in 1540, following an Act of Parliament the Company of Barbers and Surgeons was formed by merging The Fellowship of Surgeons with The Barbers Company. The association between the two was probably no more than the fact that they both used sharp knives. Two hundred years later, in 1745, the surgeons broke away to form the Company of Surgeons, which became The Royal College of Surgeons in 1800. In 1843, with a new Royal Charter it became, as it is now, The Royal College of Surgeons of England.

Again, there are Royal Colleges in Edinburgh (the oldest) and Ireland and the combined one in Glasgow. One must be a Fellow, by examination, of one or more of these Royal Colleges to practice as a surgeon in Ireland and the UK.

Another, slightly confusing, historical concept is that of the Apothecaries, but they could be thought of as the forerunners of what evolved into the General Practitioners.

They prepared and sold medicinal substances and in 1617 a Worshipful Society of Apothecaries of London was founded by Royal Charter. Their professional status was enhanced in 1704 when The House of Lords confirmed that they could prescribe and dispense medications. In 1815 The Apothecaries Act allowed them to conduct examinations and issue licences.

The whole process of teaching, licencing and regulating medical practice in England was haphazard through the late 17th, 18th and 19th centuries and lagged noticeably behind Scotland. The gradual transfer of hospital care from the church to the philanthropic evolved into the establishment of three types of hospital; the Voluntary, the Municipal and the Cottage. The most prestigious were the Voluntary, where the philanthropy was based on historical prestige and charitable endowments. The most important of these were the Teaching hospitals, of which 10 of the 22 were in London. There were about 1000 other non-teaching Voluntaries spread around the UK. None of the Hospital Medical Schools was attached to a university until the 18th century and by the 19th century England, certainly, was falling behind the USA and continental European countries like Germany in terms of medical teaching and research.

The first UK University Medical School was established in Edinburgh in1726, followed by Glasgow in 1744. In England, the first to incorporate with London University was St. Georges in 1751. Many of the "great" London Teaching Hospitals vehemently resisted what they perceived as a loss of independence for their Medical Schools, but in 1858 The Medical Act was passed resulting in the creation of The General Medical Council and The Medical Register. Even Oxford, where "Physic" had been taught from the 13th century and Viscount Nuffield had endowed the five clinical chairs of medicine and surgery (including the 1st Professor of Anaesthetics and the 2nd Professor of Orthopaedics in the world) in the 1930's, only created a Medical School in 1946. Cambridge, where medicine had been taught since 1540, did not create their Medical School until 1976.

The Municipal Hospitals had existed scattered around the country from the 18th century, but they really appeared in numbers after the industrial revolution and into the 19th century. Their philanthropic support was civic pride but there was no real interest in teaching, they were considered as the poor relations of the Voluntary hospitals. They provided a combination of social and medical care; I suspect that the voluntary hospitals were constantly trying to discharge patients for whom they felt they had nothing further to offer to the municipal. This practice continues between the Specialist Units of the teaching hospitals and the District General Hospitals today. There would be resident medical and surgical staff and other specialists could be asked to attend.

The Cottage Hospitals were entrepreneurial institutions serving a smaller, more intimate community. They would be run by nursing staff and served medically by the GPs, that group of doctors "descended" from the apothecaries, who had chosen to specialise, not in a particular aspect of medicine or surgery, but in a community.

The three types did not get on well.

They neither liked nor trusted each other and constantly suspected the others of trying to take advantage of them. The Voluntaries, for instance, put a lot of effort into their outpatient clinics which the others could not do because they did not have the staff. The Municipals resented this because it was a source of patients and prestige and the GP's resented it because it was their principal (only?) source of income.

Towards the end of the eighteenth century the concept of a "welfare state" began to emerge. This is often associated with Thomas Paine, an English born American writer and radical thinker. In 1791 and 1792 he published, in two parts, *Rights of Man* in which he strongly supported the French revolution, although it was beginning to descend into the bloody carnage which came to be known as The Reign of Terror. In the book he describes a mechanism for creating a welfare state in Britain, although he probably did not coin the term, which included the abolition of The Monarchy. The book was widely read before it was banned, when he returned to France. He was tried as a traitor *in absentia* and condemned to death. Very wisely, he never returned to England. He was more interested in social justice and the redistribution of wealth than healthcare, though his concepts of provision of care for the elderly and infirm were central to his welfare beliefs. He died in New York in 1809, and thus lived for ten years to observe the unstable oligarchy, which replaced The Monarchy in France, progress into the outright Dictatorship of The Emperor Napoleon, whose principal objective was to subjugate, through military might, as much of the world as possible. To achieve this, he was prepared to enslave entire nations and introduce a *Levee en masse*, forced conscription into the army (so much for *Liberte, Egalite, Fraternite)*. Clearly, much of Paine's thinking was a little flawed but the concept of a welfare state had been seeded and by the middle of the nineteenth century there was increasing political interest in state provision of healthcare. In the UK The National Insurance Act of 1911, largely the work of David Lloyd George the Liberal Chancellor, was a political forerunner to what became the National Health Service.

Aneurin Bevan was born in South Wales, in 1897. He left school at 13 and went to work as a miner, where he quickly became involved in local union politics. At 19 he was named head of his Miners Lodge, he joined the Labour party and attended the Central Labour College in London where, apparently, he was not a particularly outstanding or enthusiastic student. On returning to South Wales, he could find no employment for three years until he became a union official. He was an active figure in the 1926 General Strike. In 1929, he was elected as the Member of Parliament for Ebbw Vale (his successor was Michael Foot). He quickly set the tone for his political life, becoming an enthusiastic critic of numerous politicians from all parties. During the war he was particularly vociferous against Winston Churchill and the wartime government, basically adopting the stance that Britain should align itself more with Russia and take less interest in involving the United States in the struggle. Clement Attlee formed a Labour government following their victory in the post-war 1945 general election. He had a large majority and was able to embark on an ambitious programme of social reforms, as outlined in their manifesto, which became dubbed the 'Welfare State'. He appointed Bevan as the Minister of Health with a remit to cover housing. At the age of 47 he was the youngest member of Attlee's Cabinet and although he was described by The Times as "an outstanding back bench critic" he had a history of disciplinary problems within the Labour Party itself and his appointment was considered something of a surprise. Attlee, however, said that he was "starting with me with a clean sheet" and his brief was basically to create the National Health Service.

In some respects, comparing him to more recent Labour politicians, Nye Bevan sounds like an obstreperous

Welsh combination of John Prescott and Jeremy Corbyn, but as Minister of Health in the immediate post-war years he was undoubtedly the perfect selection. He was possessed of strong Celtic passion and a true and unshakable compassion. He had been inspired by the Tredegar Medical Aid Society in his hometown in South Wales and others such as the earlier Great Western Railway Medical Aid Society in Swindon. He had served on committees overseeing the management of cottage hospitals and health services by local authorities. He was in the right place as Minister of Health in a government with a large enough majority to pursue many of the reforms described in its pre-election manifesto, and in pursuing his own brief to create a National Health Service he relished attempts at intimidation by numerous politicians from both sides of the house and the British Medical Association. Having been involved in the management of Unions from the age of 19, I doubt if he was overly impressed by the medical professions attempt to form a union of its own.

Also, he was fortunate that it was the right time for such reform. Bevan and Attlee's Labour government were credited with the foundation of the National Health Service, but I doubt if it could have happened if there had not been a groundswell of public opinion that this was the right thing to do. After "the war to end all wars", the General Strike and the Great Depression, and a desperate struggle for very survival in the Second World War (apart from some civilian bombing in the Spanish Civil War the Second World War was the first to involve civilians on a massive scale) even the most reactionary of politicians must have felt that the subjects of The UK deserved some reward for their endurance, so Bevan's National Health Service Act was passed in 1946 and came into force, as planned, on 5th July 1948.

Bevan had courage and integrity. Winston Churchill, who had described him during the war as "a squalid nuisance", later observed that he was "one of the few members that I will sit still and listen to". In the time between the passing of the NHS Act and its coming into force Bevan said, "all I am doing is extending to the entire population of Britain the benefits we had in Tredegar for a generation or more". He later wrote "no society can legitimately call itself civilised if a sick person is denied medical aid because of lack of means". That remains an absolute truism that should always be applied to the provision of health care, but it is also very usefully vague. It is impossible to know, in medical terms, precisely what Bevan meant by the word "sick" and even today that remains one of the NHS's greatest difficulties. In terms of Bevan's intentions, the only absolute certainty is that the British government should pick up the bill. The concept of "free at the time of need" or "free at the point of delivery" remains the central pillar of public thinking, but perhaps that is no longer universally appropriate in the twenty first century. It is difficult now for us to recall the very limited extent of medical interventions in the 1940s and '50s, just as it would have been impossible for anyone involved in health care then to imagine the degree of complexity and diversity of investigations and interventions which are now considered to be a minimum standard for health care; and which are often frighteningly expensive.

So, what can we learn from history? What did post-mediaeval society understand from the word "sick"? If the changes in health care over the lifetime of the NHS are incredible how much more incredible are the changes of every aspect of life from the 16th century to the 21st. There is no point in considering the differences, but it is worth reflecting on the similarities between what was considered optimal health care from the 16th to the 19th centuries and what the NHS should be aspiring to provide. In those days they may not have had much of an armamentarium for treating the sick, just physical and emotional care – what we would call "nursing". Today the first essential for good health care delivery is, of course, good quality nursing care. In that period, they began to understand the nature of infectious diseases and a young physician in Bristol is credited with developing the first ever vaccine. How important has that become to us today! They assumed responsibility for the infirm, the aged, the homeless, the destitute. This is social welfare, not Tom Paine's brain-dead economic welfare state where everybody is poor so as not to risk the unfair possibility of some people being relatively rich; this is what the NHS should be empowered to assume responsibility for.

In the 18th and 19th centuries they cared, in their own way, for the mentally ill. We may now consider the way they did it as barbaric, but at least they tried. They tried not to let them starve, homeless in the gutter. There was considerable debate in1947 as to whether the NHS should take responsibility for the mentally ill; of course it should. We must try and there is nothing better than the NHS to try, but I bet that in 100 years our treatment of mental illness will be considered utterly inhumane. Knowing that our efforts will be ridiculed by future generations we should not scorn the attempts of past generations to do the best they could, based on the beliefs and concepts of their society at that time.

We must also look back in time to consider what the NHS has done well up to now and what it does rather poorly, then try to identify why there are those failings.

It is, and has been for several decades, a good medical disaster and emergency service. I think of a medical disaster as a manageable but probably incurable long term potentially fatal illness. If, for the moment, we exclude malignant disease, cancer in all its forms, this would include conditions such as renal failure, diabetes, ischemic heart disease and heart failure, chronic respiratory conditions and afflictions of the digestive tract including liver failure.

But there is a second group of potentially disastrous diseases for which management and care in the fairly recent past has not been of a particularly high standard. These are neurological disorders such as stroke, or progressive degenerative disorders of the central nervous system such as dementia, or peripheral nervous system such as motor neurone disease and, perhaps above all, would be mental illness.

It is interesting to speculate why there should have been this dichotomy within the service. I do not think it is due to any different commitment from the various specialists treating these conditions, but rather that our understanding of them remains very primitive. In the eighteenth century it was standard practice to bleed a patient with a fever, this induced a degree of hypovolaemic shock which corrected the principal observable symptom – hot skin. It also caused faintness and sweating, which were thought to be good symptoms of a response. Today we know that it was the worst thing that could have been done and it probably killed a great many people; yet electro-convulsive therapy (basically a massive electric shock to the brain administered under controlled anaesthesia) is still used in the management of depression; it may improve mood, but I doubt if it treats the underlying cause.

So, for this second group of patients we have extraordinarily little in the way of diagnostic tests or therapeutic interventions. Developments in imaging and interventional radiology are beginning to make great improvements in stroke management and medical geneticists are giving some insights in diagnosis but there is often little or nothing, as yet, in the way of treatment. I suspect that this inadequacy was driven, at least in part, by society, which seems to have forgotten that degeneration and death are the inevitable sequelae of life. Those patients within the first group will die from their condition, probably in hospital and perhaps in circumstances of tragedy for their family and friends. This is considered unacceptable and so receives a great deal of funding and attention. The patients in the second group probably will not die from their condition in an acute way, although their quality of life may deteriorate and they may well ultimately die, hidden away in a care home, as a result of their underlying pathological condition. This is not considered to be an unacceptable tragedy however unacceptable the quality of life may be to the victim of the condition. The exception is mental illness which can lead directly to suicide, or murder, an acute and tragic event. Perhaps for this reason mental health is now coming to the forefront of public attention, but I see little increased interest in the management of progressive neurological disabilities such as Parkinson's disease.

There is nothing to suggest that this double standard of clinical interest is unique to the United Kingdom, but if we are truly to have the best healthcare delivery system in the world (and there is no reason why we should not) then this double standard should be overcome.

That brings me to consider cancer, that most emotive of all diseases. I use the term not in its pathologically correct sense but in the sense of its public perception; that is all forms of malignantly progressive aberrant growths that can spread throughout the body and are ultimately fatal. The progress made in the last thirty years in the management of all cancers (some, of course, more than others) is truly astonishing. It has been made possible by just that very emotive nature of the disease; cancer is extremely well funded for research and resourced for its management. That, in a way, is right and proper; we should pay the most attention to the things that most concern us; but it shows what can be achieved, particularly in the field of research. On the whole cancers are managed well by the NHS; no one is denied treatment, although some treatments are denied in some cases. This is sometimes picked up by relatives and the press as being "cost driven", but the reality is nearly always simply that the treatment has no chance of being successful. It is very sad to see families and friends throwing large sums of money and false hopes at clinicians, often in other countries, offering expensive therapeutic interventions which are not sanctioned by the NHS. The reason they are not sanctioned is nearly always because there is no scientific basis for thinking that they might confer any lasting benefit.

The media also seems addicted to stories of poorer survival rates in this country compared to other comparable socio-economic nations. International comparisons are fraught with potential errors in classification and differing interpretations, but it does seem that we could have better outcomes if there was earlier diagnosis. Many of the subclassifications of tumours and the therapeutic options for their treatment have been developed in this country, but it is difficult to apply them if one does not have early access to the patients. This has now become a very hot topic, thanks to the altered priorities of health care imposed by the pandemic.

Another thing that, by and large, is done extremely well is the management of acute trauma. Sometimes this is life threatening such as severe road traffic accidents or stabbings; sometimes it is basically just an inconvenience, such as a simple broken bone. This, overall, is treated efficiently, promptly and successfully. For broken bones, however, there are exceptions which again involve the people whose life is not obviously going to be immediately changed by the fracture. These are people whose quality of life is already dramatically diminished by some co-morbidity, the most common of which is senility. It does also tend to be the case with people who have other severe disabilities whatever their age. For instance, hip fractures in the elderly are a common and quite frequently terminal event. Although outcomes have improved somewhat it remains the case that they are often internally fixed or treated by some form of hip replacement on an "out of hours" operating list for emergencies and performed by relatively junior trainees. Their rehabilitation, if they survive the operation, and their discharge planning may be perfunctory at best.

Inevitably, from the point of view of care quality, there are regional variations and variations between hospitals within the same locality. If I required surgery, say for a broken limb, I can think of hospitals and surgeons whom I would not choose to undertake a major procedure; but, for better or worse, that type of "inside" information is not widely available to the general public.

There is also an inevitable differing response within the same clinical team to different challenges. The unusual and dramatic is exciting, but the commonplace and banal is mundane and receives less attention. This is human nature and can never really be completely eliminated, probably nor should it be.

Another important consideration is to remember what any therapeutic intervention is attempting to achieve. All treatment options for any situation range from doing nothing, perhaps because nothing other than reassurance is needed, to undertaking a procedure which will inevitably leave the patient worse off than they were prior to the intervention. Sometimes it is appropriate to do nothing even where the presenting condition will inevitably be fatal. If, in any intervention, we subject a terminally ill or injured patient to more distress with no change in their quality or duration of life, or relief of pain, then it is better to do nothing and simply keep them comfortable.

It can be exceedingly difficult, perhaps even impossible, for a family to accept that no "heroic intervention" is truly in the best interests of the patient. Sometimes such treatments are forced upon the clinical team by the family, particularly in the case of untreatable tumours in children. This must be an incredibly difficult situation to manage, I suppose the overriding principle must simply be damage limitation for all involved.

Another group of clinical conditions are those that require elective surgery. This is a situation where a disease process is affecting the quality of life of the patient, but is in no way life threatening, and the main problem facing the NHS for this situation is that of the famous waiting lists. I think I show, in the next chapter, that this has been more a perceived problem than a real one and there are ways of dealing with it effectively.

A much more significant problem facing the NHS than waiting lists is care of the elderly and disabled. The dysfunctional relationship between acute or sub-acute medical care, rehabilitation and long-term social care is a problem that absolutely must be resolved. Bed-blocking is a term used to describe the situation where a patient is safely past the need for relatively high dependency nursing care, let alone daily medical input or review, but is still occupying an acute hospital bed because there is nowhere to transfer them where they can be comfortably and safely well cared for; either until they are fit to return to their family or home, or for the rest of their lives. It goes without saying that acute care is massively more expensive than rehabilitation or social care and bed-blocking is probably the commonest cause of "same day" cancellations of planned elective operations or investigations. These cancellations are really horrible for the patients and their families and are also hugely expensive; an operating theatre or a sophisticated imaging devise staffed and ready to go but lying idle because the patient had to be sent home is almost criminally stupid.

Lip service is paid to schemes like "integrated care pathways" and "discharge planning" but in fact there is very little that is integrated or planned; there are simply too many variables.

Perhaps the NHS should assume control of all social and disability care. From cradle to grave, its remit and its power should be enlarged and strengthened, not sold off piecemeal to private enterprise.

But assuming control is not the same thing as "blank cheque" funding, there could be dignified private accommodation for everybody without cost at the point of delivery. Then, if an individual or their family wanted to pay a bit more for some extra facility, like a private sitting room or a spare bedroom, let them do so; they might well share them with friends they had made in the same community. There will always be inequalities of wealth within society but that is not necessarily a bad thing.

Nye Bevan himself said, thinking about housing when he was Secretary of State for Health "we should try to introduce in our modern villages and towns what was always the lovely feature of English and Welsh villages where the doctor, the grocer, the butcher and the farm labourer, all lived in the same street. I believe that it is essential for the full life of citizens to see the living tapestry of a mixed community." That is a very astute observation. We seem to have lost that a bit as a nation, but there is no reason why it should not be reintroduced to the environment of a care home.

From a patient's perspective probably the biggest difficulty with the NHS is "Access". This is the firewall that threatens to overwhelm the service; the desperate fight to match supply to the increasingly strident and impatient demand. Days, or even weeks, to get to see a general practitioner. Hours, or even days, to be seen and treated in an Accident and Emergency Department. Uncertainty and delay in hospital appointments and treatment.

Within the NHS the biggest problem, in my opinion, is collapsing morale. It is tiring and very depressing to be constantly fighting a losing battle against a firewall.

Yet the NHS does many things very well. Most of the perceived failings are structural and organisational rather than simple "underfunding".

Each of these failings is amenable to some type of solution and I hope, in this short book, to address the greatest of them in turn.

To paraphrase Bevan from earlier in this chapter; if a civilised society is one that protects the weak, then it must have a satisfactory state health care delivery service.

It should also support knowledge, freedom of speech and the arts and in protecting the weak it must acknowledge the value of the strong.

The NHS should be a beacon and a cornerstone for the values of our society, but it must adapt to provide good and inclusive health care for all in the 21st Century.

Chapter 2

The NHS as an employer; is it worth saving?

Between the passing of the National Health Service Act in 1946, and its implementation on 5th July 1948, the British Medical Association, described Aneurin Bevan as "a complete and uncontrolled dictator", dubbed him the "Tito of Tonypandy" and threatened to derail the National Health Service scheme before it had even begun. After eighteen months of dispute Bevan finally won them over by making some minor concessions including allowing consultants to keep their own private practices, but he did not compromise the fundamental principles of his NHS proposals. Later in describing how he managed to broker the deal he famously claimed that "I stuffed their mouths with gold". I guess we will never know what he really meant by this. It may have been intended as a witty or dismissive response to a question, it might have been an angry conclusion to eighteen frustrating months, or it might be that his only significant non-political employment, ever, had been a few years in his teens as a coal miner and, on that basis, he regarded a doctor's income as unimaginable gold. Whatever lay behind the remark, having worked, albeit many years later, in the NHS for forty years, I cannot believe that more than a handful of clinicians would respond simply to a giant payoff. I think it is important to remember the saying (which could also be applied to politicians) that doctors are like manure – spread thinly they can be useful but put them all in a heap and they stink. The BMA may have been fighting a phantasm in a battle that they could not, in any case, win and gradually individual doctors and other clinicians came to realise that Bevan's proposals were truly the way forwards for a health care delivery system.

Whatever the truth was at that time, I believe that the majority of the UK's population over the last sixty years would feel that the principal motivation of clinicians within the NHS was to be of service to their community, not primarily (I admit there are a few rather offensive exceptions) to pursue personal financial gain.

The English have a bizarre misconception of the meaning of the word service. I cannot really answer for the other three devolved nations but in England people seem to consider that to be of service is in some way demeaning; in fact, to be of service is the highest achievement to which any individual can aspire. The French understand this, and I use the word in its true sense. It is a pity that governments, over many years, have forgotten that their role is not to rule the people but to serve them.

For many years (certainly in my lifetime) the NHS has only survived on the good will of its workforce, but over the last decade or more that goodwill has been leaching away pretty fast. The NHS is probably now perceived by most of its employees as a bad employer. That is certainly true of the frontline workers. Successive governments have cynically exploited the knowledge that clinicians, by their own beliefs and commitments, are immensely reluctant to take any form of industrial action. The consequence of this is that in the general scramble for improved standards of living the clinicians in the NHS have been increasingly left behind and in real terms salaries have diminished significantly over the last twenty years. But it is not just the money which is the reason why morale amongst the NHS workforce is now so low – it is also the conditions.

All frontline workers could earn more money working elsewhere than in the NHS. Secretaries are fixed on ridiculously low bandings whilst undertaking hugely responsible and difficult tasks. The manual workers (porters, cleaners, maintenance staff, etc) have all worked within the NHS because of the variety of the job and the feeling of being part of a community. That is just no longer the case and most of them are becoming increasingly unlikely to persevere within the service. Porters and cleaners have been sold off to commercial firms that make a profit out of them and treat them even worse than the NHS would. Maintenance work has often been taken over, incredibly inefficiently and at huge expense, by the appalling so called Private Finance Initiative (PFI) Partners, a sort of privatisation for financing new buildings. The sense of being valued and appreciated as somebody who contributes to their community by working for the NHS has gradually been eroded by a variety of socio-economic factors, but it remains an important incentive for continuing within that employment. The relatively brief surge of "pandemic emotion" will not change that in the long term.

There are numerous other reasons why The NHS is no longer regarded as a good employer and these will be dealt with appropriately in subsequent specific chapters. The basic point is that the NHS no longer shows any care and consideration for its workforce. Perhaps it has just become too large an organisation to "give a little of that human touch". It may be true that increasing size brings some benefits, but it also creates an impersonal feeling of worthlessness. There is no reason why, within specific units of the organisation, individuals should not continue to feel valued and cared for; but that is not The NHS way, as will be discussed.

If the NHS is as poor an employer as I believe it to be that brings me to the question in this chapter's title; is it actually worth saving? After all, no country in the world (except perhaps Norway, which has a unique combination of huge natural resources, a very small population and a highly enlightened government) has both the financial power and the willingness within government to provide universal health care for its entire population, so why should the UK attempt to? Despite the seeming impossibility of a moderately wealthy country like the UK funding a free to all at the point of delivery optimal health care system, the answer to the question "should the NHS be saved" is, as I hope to show, very emphatically yes.

The habit of the nation, for several decades now, has been to complain about the NHS. The "let down by the NHS" syndrome is enhanced by the media who glorify in taking a swipe at it at every opportunity. Stories of individuals' personal distress, pain, disability or poor outcome are presented by the media with nauseating frequency and relish. National panics about things like waiting times, hospital hygiene, infection rates, and cancer care are promulgated with glee in the press and on television.

In a material sense it has always been natural within our culture for people to value most of all the things for which they feel some sense of ownership. In the eyes of the public, I believe that the NHS has become just an amorphous "right". A part of the state's responsibility to care for them in every way, with a system for which they feel no personal involvement and a cause for justifiable complaint if they feel let down in any way.

The reality is that the NHS performs very well compared to other nations' health care delivery systems. The following data come from published studies, all by international groups or organisations like The World Health Organisation, The Commonwealth Fund, International Health Policy Surveys and OECD Health between the period of 2011 – 2014. That is a little out of date, but precise contemporaneous data are hard to come by and in any case that period coincides with a high level of public dissatisfaction with the NHS. They were brought to my attention in a paper given to a private society which is in my Acknowledgements. I have chosen six reports, slightly simplified and presented as text to show only the data relevant to this discussion.

1. The NHS has been cited as the largest single employer in Europe. If that is the case it does not apply to doctors. A publication in 2014 of practicing physicians per 100,000 inhabitants in each European country shows the United Kingdom to be about comparable with Slovenia and Romania, rather less than Serbia and Macedonia, and just a little bit more

than Montenegro, Turkey and Poland. Successive governments have promised to employ more doctors, but I do not see much sign of that. It takes about ten years to train a doctor. This must be addressed, but I acknowledge that there is no simple, single solution.

2. A study of total health expenditure per capita shows the USA to be the biggest by far with about 50% private and 50% public. The UK is about the same as New Zealand and Italy with about one sixth of the total being private, which is one of the lowest proportions amongst the affluent countries of the world. It is just over one third of that of the USA and just over one half of that of Norway, but it is noticeably less than France, Germany and Australia. My conclusion is that it is pretty cost effective.

3. Looking at purely public health expenditure the US falls to third behind Norway at the top and then the Netherlands. The UK is just in the bottom half and above Australia, Finland, Ireland and New Zealand. However, if you include private expenditure all four of these countries come out higher than the UK. It is of course important to remember that public health expenditure is a very blunt way of evaluating a nation's commitment to its health care delivery, but it shows that performance "free at the point of delivery" is particularly good in the UK.

4. In a study about cost related barriers to accessing health care, data were expressed as a percentage of people who experienced access barriers due to costs, over the course of one year. That is defined as people who did not fill or take their prescriptions, did not

visit a doctor with a medical problem and/or did not receive the care recommended; put simply, the patients did not get what they needed. This is a study of only eight countries. The worst performing nation was the USA at 37%, the Netherlands were 22% and New Zealand 21%. The last two figures surprise me, the first does not. Australia, which is largely a slightly less grasping version of the American model, was 16% and Canada 13%. Norway was 10% and Sweden 6% - both these figures are a surprise, but, no surprise, the UK was the lowest (i.e., the best performing) at 4%. This shows that higher expenditure does not correspond directly to patients getting their intended care.

5. This study and the previous one, are, to some extent, soft outcome studies. That is to say they, at least in part, rely on patients' subjective responses to questions, just as a predictive political opinion poll deals in voters' responses to questions. Nevertheless, they both deal in what are broadly termed Patient Related Outcome Measures which are currently a very widely accepted way of evaluating healthcare delivery outcomes. They have their weaknesses and no doubt one day will fall out of favour, but at the moment (like opinion polls in politics) they are as good a way as we have of predicting what will happen or evaluating what has happened. In this study seven European countries, two northern hemisphere countries and two southern hemisphere countries were ranked according to a number of criteria. These were; "quality of care" considered as effective care,

safe care, co-ordinated care, and patient-centred care; "access" meaning cost related problems and timeliness of care; "equity" meaning essentially fairness and impartiality of the service; and "healthy lives" meaning the background health status of the overall population of the nation. So, the ranking for each of the 11 nations in each of the criteria was evaluated at 1 – 11, with 11 being bottom, the worst. The US came eleventh in four considerations but one of them was the background health of the nation, which is obviously a difficulty in providing a satisfactory health care service. Norway, very surprisingly, came bottom in quality of care and seventh in co-ordinated care. I think this illustrates the dangers of some of these soft outcome evaluations; perhaps the Norwegians just have very unrealistic expectations. France came bottom in access overall, scoring tenth in cost-related problems and timeliness of care, it also scored tenth in patient-centred care. Sweden, again surprisingly, came tenth in quality of care scoring ten in effective care and eleven in co-ordinated care. Canada came bottom in timeliness of care, no surprise as they have banned all private provision, and scored tenth in safe care and efficiency. Germany was tenth in co-ordinated care. New Zealand was tenth in equity and the UK was tenth in the health of the nation. Some of these bottom two positions are quite surprising to me, but sadly not second worst for UKs overall health, a reflection of our increasing problem with obesity. Australia, the Netherlands and Switzerland were not placed in the bottom two for anything. The really striking outcome however is that the UK was ranked third out of the eleven for timeliness of care and second for equity. For everything else it was ranked one, the best. The overall rankings from top to bottom were UK best, then Switzerland. Sweden, Australia, Germany and the Netherlands tied third, New Zealand and Norway tied seventh, France ninth, Canada tenth and the US at the bottom, eleventh. This suggests that by far the highest expenditure can still lead to clearly the worst provision of care.

6.   The final study I want to describe looked at the waiting period in days for surgery of the knee and hip, the vast majority of which will be elective procedures. It looked at a rather random selection of thirteen countries around the world and the UK was rated third best at just under one hundred days. Shorter than that were Denmark and the Netherlands. This was less time than New Zealand, Norway, Spain and Portugal but it may be significant that the USA, France, Germany, Australia, and Switzerland were not included in this study. My conclusion is that waiting times in The UK for elective surgery may actually be among the best in the world, especially for a nation with such a low proportion of practicing physicians and spending so little on private care.

Anyone in the UK who has followed the management of the coronavirus pandemic should have realised that, in a medical context, science is not an exact science. I am sure that somebody who wished to could produce a whole series of other outcome studies to show that the NHS is not performing particularly well, but we have also learned from the pandemic that different countries have different ways of collecting their data and probably also that some countries just point-blank lie.

My own absolute conviction is that, with a comparatively exceedingly small number of clinicians per head of population and a relatively low expenditure, the NHS is performing fantastically well. Individual patients or specific individual communities will continue to be "let down" by individual clinicians or groups of clinicians whether the healthcare is being delivered in the public or the private environment. Indeed, it is my absolute certainty that poor care is more prevalent in the private environment than in the NHS, which I discuss in Chapter 10.

I feel entirely justified in the very firm conclusion that, quite apart from moral and ethical considerations and the desire to be part of a "civilised society", a national health system is by far the most efficient, effective, and compassionate way of delivering health care to a nation.

Jennie Lee was a Scottish socialist who was elected as a Labour MP from 1929 to 1931, at the time the youngest female member of the House. She was, possibly, even more of a firebrand than Bevan himself. They married in1934 and she was a considerable influence on his political career. She was returned to parliament in Labour's land-slide victory of 1945 and after Bevan's death from stomach cancer in 1960 (aged 62) went on to a long and distinguished career in public service, being ennobled as Baroness Lee of Asheridge, serving in Harold Wilson's government and, amongst other achievements, playing a key role in the formation of the Open University.

She said "Of course the health service did not begin in 1948. Many of us have associations with the between-the-wars health service; a great patchwork, a good deal of good intentions, a great deal of inadequacies".

The formation of the NHS was the best chance of unifying the service and addressing those inadequacies.

With a bit of re-thinking our National Health Service could easily be much better, perhaps even deserving of the slightly fatuous, but highly gratifying, epithet of "the envy of the world".

The NHS must be saved.

Chapter 3

What is NHS Management; Why is it failing?

I should open this chapter by saying that just as clinicians feel hamstrung by an outmoded and inefficient organisation, it may well be that many NHS managers and strategists feel that they are suffering under the same burden. It is however an inescapable fact that there is a very unhealthy relationship between the managers and the clinicians. The doctors believe they have been saddled with poor managers and the managers regard doctors as unmanageable. There is some truth in both attitudes.

Most of the managers that I have had personal dealings with were reasonably capable and well-motivated people, doing their best in a difficult job, with genuine concern and compassion for the patients. The Medical Directors that I worked for in my own hospital were all personal friends, which is not quite the same as saying that I always agreed with them, but it does mean that I always respected them.

I believe there are certain difficulties in strategically planning and managing a health care delivery system which are peculiar to that particular environment. One of them is, as I have previously mentioned, that so much of the evaluation of the effectiveness and efficiency of healthcare delivery is in measures of soft outcomes, which are extremely difficult to quantify. It is not like managing a manufacturing or a sales company, where success can be computed in hard figures. It is not even like the hospitality industry, where again soft outcomes are important and difficult to quantify. But a hotel's popularity can be gauged by its occupancy as well as by accounts and guest feedback. The same is true of a restaurant or a pub. These facilities however do not try to cater for everybody; indeed, they tend to subspecialise, aiming at a particular niche in the market. Some people like to base their holidays around the discos of a Mediterranean beach resort, others to go bird watching in The Outer Hebrides. Some parents like to take their children to Theme Parks, others for a walk in the country or a day on the beach. It is a matter of personal choice, but no one would choose to spend two weeks feeling ill in hospital, let alone have that inflicted upon their children.

A health care delivery service must try to fulfil the needs of an entire population, often in great distress.

What feedback it does receive is, sadly, usually in the form of complaints, most of which are gratuitously stupid and ill informed. I, for instance, was once reported to the GMC by a D-Day veteran on whom I had performed a hip replacement. The operation went fine but he was terribly angry that I had not removed a piece of shrapnel about half the size of an airgun pellet which he had had in the soft tissues around his hip since the war. He was elderly and somewhat confused and was completely unable to grasp the difference between removing a foreign body that one came upon by chance during an elective procedure and deliberately searching for an inert foreign body which was causing no problems. To search for it would have prolonged the operative procedure and jeopardised the outcome. I spent many hours explaining this to him over a period of years and always got on very well with him, but, following each consultation, after a few days, another letter of complaint would arrive demanding to know why I had not removed the piece of shrapnel. Eventually he sent one to the GMC who were obliged to inform me and investigate, before telling me that there was no case to answer. I cite this instance, not because it particularly bothered me, but because it illustrates the difficulty of dealing with that kind of complaint and the amount of time and energy that it wastes as a totally useless piece of feedback.

Most important of all however, is that a health care delivery system cannot, it certainly should not, be seeking to gain popularity on the basis of how comfortable or luxurious it is. Sadly, the general public have no feedback themselves to distinguish between truly effective high-quality clinical care and the worthless value of luxury accommodation in a clinical situation.

Remember that most of the patients of the late Dr Harold Shipman described him as the perfect GP, until he murdered them.

Basically, trying to manage a healthcare system is infinitely more difficult than trying to manage a hotel, run a pub, or be the chief executive officer of an airline or a manufacturing company.

Another problem that strategists and managers have is that they are caught between a rock and a hard place. The hard place is the fact that if developments continue to be made in the field of investigation and treatment of diseases, then the ensuing costs will also increase. That is never going to change, and I do not think any of us would wish it to. As

Bevan himself predicted in 1948, the NHS will always be overspent. The rock of course is basically the politicians. However desperate the politicians are to gain favour with the electorate, the reality is that the funding is finite. Within the current structure that cannot be changed.

To make matters worse, it is generally believed amongst the frontline workers, probably rightly, that the managers salary structures are linked to bonuses for monetary savings which are usually achieved at the expense of clinical services, masquerading as improved efficiency. This just means that the clinicians and the front line that supports them must work even harder to maintain the same level of clinical care and service. Not a good basis for a working relationship.

I hope I have defined, reasonably simply and clearly, what I mean by a clinician or a frontline worker, but I find it much harder to explain what I mean by the term "manager". I suppose the simplest way is to say that it is anyone on the NHS payroll who is not a frontline worker. Another way of expressing that is to include anyone whose job description does not involve, regularly and routinely, direct one to one communication with a patient, either face to face or electronically by email or telephone. Thus, a ward clerk or appointments clerk is not a manager, they have a key clinical role (although by my definition they are not "clinicians") in putting a patient or their relatives minds at ease; but an IT specialist who organises and maintains the computer systems is.

Similarly, a porter pushing a patient in a wheelchair to Xray, or on their bed to the operating theatre can chat to and help relax a patient at a time that might be very stressful for them – the good ones do, which is why they enjoy their jobs. The head porter might enjoy helping out his team by regularly pushing beds, many do because they enjoy a clinical role, but if they only sit in their office and issue instructions, they are a manager. I have no problem with that, it may well be the best way in which they can contribute to the efficient running of the organisation, which makes them, as a manager, a valuable member of the team.

The difficulty which I am trying to illustrate is that clinicians and front-line workers may have to "manage" situations, while many "managers" will choose, for whatever reason, to take on a frontline role from time to time.

It becomes even more complicated when trying to describe the structure and hierarchy of the management group. The first tier is the supervisor; these can usually be identified by their "badge" of the clipboard. They are essentially collectors of data. Often, they are clinicians or front liners whose career structure has drawn them into a management role in order to enhance their salary; they may well not really like it, but money talks. Examples would be the nurse who has taken on the role of theatre manager or bed manager, or the cleaner who has taken on the role of supervisor (quality control). I was always rather depressed by the frequency with which patients observed, in passing, that they saw more cleaning supervisors with clipboards than cleaners with cleaning equipment.

These are in the "administrator" group, whose responsibilities increase from data collection to organisation.

The next tier is the "manager" group, whose responsibilities start at organisation but rise to the level of strategic planning. They may have started life as clinicians, I have a special place in my mind for this group, or they may have gone into NHS Management directly from school or university or the commercial/industrial world. This is the largest group, for the sake of clarity, this is probably the group I have most often in mind whenever I refer to management or managers.

The final tier is the pure strategists, the planners, organisational details are beneath their intellectual visionary status. These may be drawn from the most successful of the managing former clinicians, but often they are the great and the good who have been distinguished, for good or bad, in other walks of life. In so far as he had a strategic role in the NHS this, to everyone's shame, is the group that Jimmy Saville would have fitted into. More well intentioned, certainly not evil, this is also where the politicians enter the picture.

The strategists can function at a local/regional level or at a national level, where the politicians have the greatest power because they hold the purse-strings. The logical conclusion to this would seem to be that the chief strategist is The Secretary of State for Health; not exactly a position that one could regard as being a long-term job or having a great degree of continuity. There were seven Ministers of Health in the first ten years of the NHS.

The following is a story which illustrates, perfectly, the function and thinking of the different tiers of management. It is attributed to the late Labour MP Tony Benn.

The NHS held a boat race against a Japanese crew and after Japan won by a mile, a working party found the winners had eighteen people rowing and one steering while the NHS had eighteen steering and one rowing. So, the NHS spent £5 million on consultants, forming a restructured crew of four assistant steering managers, three deputy managers and a Director of Steering Services. The rower was given an incentive to row harder. They held another race and lost by two miles. So, the NHS fired the rower for poor performance, sold the boat and used the proceeds to pay a bonus to the Director of Steering Services.

This is not just a highly intelligent man being witty, it is a profound insight into the way in which NHS managers think.

The strategists of tier 3 will have decided, in their unaccountable way, that a boat race was a good thing for the NHS. Perhaps one of them had recently had an enjoyable trip to Japan or read an article about the number of Japanese athletes who had ever taken part in the University Boat Race. There have not been many (if any) so the implication would be that the NHS would compare better against Japan than, for instance, Germany, Holland, USA, Canada, Australia etc.

The managers in the upper echelons of tier 2 will have been instructed to organise and prepare for the race although they have not the faintest idea what that entails, or how to have the best chance of achieving a satisfactory outcome. They will be very uncomfortable with this because a "two horse race" will almost certainly result in a hard outcome, a dead heat being extremely unlikely. Hard outcomes are difficult to fudge.

The result is not what the strategists were expecting so they decide to throw enough money at the project to commission a Management Consultancy for advice. The managers arrange this but are naturally keen to ensure that the consultancies conclusions do not make them appear totally inept, so they instruct the upper echelons of the administrators to advise the consultants on the problems pertinent to boat racing in a health care environment. On considering those specific problems it is agreed that steering is the key to success, although that had originally been a random supposition.

Conclusion, re-structure the steering systems.

The result is now irrelevant because one of the strategists, following a conversation over lunch at The Garrick, has realised that the ability to make a boat go through water fast in the right direction has no bearing on health care delivery. Everybody, except the rower, feels pleased with themselves because it has been an excellent strategic exercise. When a real health care problem arises, a lethal pandemic for example, they will be in a much better position to deal with it.

There are real difficulties in managing a health care delivery service, I have opened this chapter by trying to explain some of them, sympathetically. But it seems to me an inescapable reality that the managers have an infinite ability to respond to repeating the same mistakes by replicating themselves and an infinitesimal ability to grasp the true cause of any given problem.

One of the biggest challenges continually facing the NHS is clinical staffing. The workforce is chronically understaffed and quite vindictively badly treated. Morale is extremely low, but management appear to do everything they can, in terms of petty and spiteful restrictions, to make the day-to-day life of the workforce as unpleasant as possible.

Little things, like withdrawing provision of refreshments for staff in a quiet area not far from their specific work location, so it is easy and quick to find them, if necessary, but away from the clinical environment and not accessible to patients. Why not give some priority to staff at food outlets; when you only have 20 minutes to grab some lunch or supper it is very frustrating to spend 19 of them in a queue of outpatients or visitors who have all the time in the world (or, if they do not, they can go elsewhere) and many of whom are likely to be morbidly obese already. I will discuss this further in later chapters but working in a modern hospital is like living in a goldfish bowl, it becomes very tiring and ultimately rather intimidating and depressing.

I can understand, from a management perspective, the advantages of having a flexible workforce, but NHS managers seem to think it is a concept they can arbitrarily impose on people with no advance notification. Clinicians with a modicum of experience have usually become quite specialised with differing elements of expertise, not to mention interest. Managers have enough insight to realise that there are clear differences amongst the doctors and there is a limit to how much they can be shunted around against their will; but they still try it occasionally. As a senior consultant I, on many occasions, had to work as my own senior house officer, but they do realise that this is counterproductive and the better among them probably see that it is potentially dangerous. They also realise that you cannot expect a physiotherapist to go and cover a day's work for an absent speech therapist. But they seem to think of nurses as being an amorphous inter-changeable mass.

Ward nurses have applied for a post on a specific unit; they would always be prepared to cover another ward in difficult circumstances, but they do not want to find themselves shunted off, with no prior notice, to a different ward every time they come into work. A theatre nurse from a gynaecology unit would be completely lost if sent to an orthopaedic theatre for the first time. For management it helps them hide their chronic staff shortages but, in their minds, it also has another more sinister advantage; everyone is left feeling lonely and vulnerable, disempowered with no sense of team identity. A classic ploy for keeping a workforce under control.

The unbelievably stupid thing is that it further exacerbates the staffing shortages because people who feel they are being bullied and taken advantage of just leave, either that Trust or The NHS altogether.

I will discuss how flexibility in the highly skilled workforce could be achieved, safely and productively in a later chapter.

The management handling of staff leave is another example of arrogance towards the clinicians. Clinicians are entitled to a certain number of days per year of so-called study leave. That is leave, to attend courses for their own professional development, which ultimately must be to the benefit of their employer. There is even supposed to be a fund to help pay for such courses but in many hospital trusts that seems to have been effectively and conveniently lost years ago. It is increasingly difficult to get study leave for both doctors and nurses, even without any help towards the cost of courses.

It is also increasingly difficult to get annual leave. Inevitably school holidays are popular in a workforce that is often relatively young with children of school age at home. The staff themselves acknowledge this within each given ward or department and it is pretty generally accepted that priority of choice should be given to people with young children, but management impose a rigidly inflexible system. What this means is that when someone applies for leave it may be turned down because there are too many other people on leave at the same time. When the leave year ends at the end of March, any leave that people have been unable to take is neither paid for nor allowed to be carried over into the next leave year. Whether or not this is actually in breach of employment law is irrelevant (although I suspect it is and if not, it should be) but, for sure, it is an incredibly stupid and short-sighted way to treat highly skilled underpaid staff who are already working hard and are in short supply.

In hospitals another huge, and growing, frustration is the difficulty of just getting to work and, once again, the management seem to have no insight into the importance of this, or how best to resolve it. Hospitals are often sited, by historical accident, at the centre of urban areas with restricted parking on site and virtually no parking in the surrounding environs.

Result, a grossly perverse interpretation of the law of supply and demand; if a commodity or facility is in limited supply, make as much money as you can from it. Parking in a hospital has been turned into a lucrative source of income for the Trusts and they apply this quite mercilessly to their own staff. If you can get a parking permit at all you have to pay an exorbitant sum for the year, with no guarantee of a space when you have paid.

The management of the parking is often sold off to a commercial parking agency and if you park "illegally" they are likely to be enthusiastic about collecting the fine. A daily rate to park for an eight-hour shift is too much, as is renting a space nearby from a local householder. Any member of staff who is deemed by the relevant management department to be on a public transport route is likely to be refused a permit to park anyway, irrespective of how long and convoluted the journey might be.

Every measure imposed by the management seems deliberately designed to make life more difficult and expensive for the frontline staff. It is almost as though the managers think they are doing people a great favour by letting them come to work at all. The old joke, about the perfect management structure for a hospital being to have no patients and thus no need to employ any clinical staff to treat them, always struck me as being too close to the truth to be amusing.

Nobody seems to have given any thought to addressing the transport problem in a creative way that could actually make life better for everyone. Why, for instance, can't they provide off site brown field parking and a regular shuttle service? It is just another manifestation of the fact that the management pay no attention to the welfare of their staff and have no insight into the importance of caring for a highly skilled workforce.

If you break it down, a health care delivery system could be relatively easy to manage. The clinicians are there to deliver clinical care with the assistance and backup of their frontline workers and the managers are there to provide the optimal environment for the delivery of that care, as well as monitoring that optimal care is being delivered. But after watching from the inside for forty years it just does not seem to work that way and I am not quite sure why.

I suppose that just as the clinicians want to treat patients, the managers want to manage people. I think they genuinely want to deliver good quality care, but the problem is, as I have said, that the judgement of good quality care can only really be made subjectively by clinicians themselves. Quangos like the Care Quality Commission can conduct inspections and make judgements, but they are only scratching the surface at best.

Things like compassion and efficiency are intangible, even good clinical outcomes can be manufactured. The ultimate hard outcome of patient care is patient death;

considered, in general, as a bad outcome. This is data which is easy to collect and to make judgements on. Some surgical specialities which provide care for a group with an inevitably high risk of death, such as cardiac surgery or neurosurgery, have their perioperative mortality rates analysed on an individual basis and made available to the public. This crude measure is open to misinterpretation in the media as "How many of their patients does this surgeon kill?".

No surgeon wants to be perceived as having a high mortality rate and the easiest way to avoid that is not to operate on patients who fall into an extra high-risk category. This has been termed "risk aversion" on the part of the surgeons and it does lead to situations where a patient is turned down for surgical treatment, thereby excluding them from what might well be, accepting a risk, the best treatment option for that patient's quality of life. In effect, it is easier to get apparently good results if you only offer surgery to patients with a simple problem and no co-morbidities.

Another way of manipulating the figures is if a patient who, effectively, dies during an operation is then maintained on life support in ITU for thirty days. On the thirty first day it ceases (in the data collection) to be a "perioperative" death and the life support can, with great regret, be withdrawn. These things may or may not happen. At best they arc just idle gossip, at worst they are incredibly rare, but it is true that good clinical practice in general goes largely unrecognised (and unrewarded) whilst callousness, inefficiency, poor non-fatal outcomes, laziness and sometimes frank deceit are ignored and unpunished by management.

A manager's desire to manage is really a wish for control, and I wonder how many NHS managers have read George Orwell's classic book *1984*; they do sometimes seem to base their principles at work on Big Brother. Orwell describes very graphically the way in which a population (or a workforce) can be controlled and manipulated by the creation of fear and distrust between individuals. Lack of communication with each other, together with the re-writing of history, prevents any group of people forming who might agree in condemning their rulers. It is a classic situation which exists in many countries in the world right now and it exists in the UK in the National Health Service.

A "blame culture" has been created in which clinicians are encouraged to report political incorrectness to the management structure. This is done by going on to the hospital's intranet and logging the supposed indiscretion electronically on a system called a Datix. This is instantly picked up and obligatorily acted upon by the managers. The reporting individual, of course, maintains their anonymity. Sadly, the Datix reports are more concerned with some perceived behavioural transgression than with anything which might influence patient welfare or safety. In fact, I have a distinct impression that truly risky clinical errors or oversights are still airbrushed by management when they are reported, unless blame can be firmly thrust upon a clinician. I give a possible example in Chapter 5 of a case where a clinician had clearly made a dangerous error, requiring, at the very least suspension pending an enquiry. But the management realised that the underlying fault lay with them for a regulatory oversight, so the case was quietly overlooked.

Another thing, perhaps the most important, that they have picked up from Orwell's nightmare scenario is the realisation that the formation of a group of people is a "team"; their collective influence is much greater than any number of individuals, so wherever possible clinicians must be made to work in isolation. People who have formed a good team trust each other and teamwork is a vital part of effective performance in every aspect of life. But teams are strong and can be difficult to control. Throughout my clinical working life, I was extraordinarily fortunate to be able to work, in the main, with people I knew and trusted, but that is becoming increasingly difficult to achieve.

In Outpatient Clinics I could be reassured that the receptionists and nursing staff would be sympathetic to the patients and effective trouble-shooters if any patient felt unhappy or hard done by. I have always believed that in an outpatient consultation with a specialist the patient needs the time it takes to have their clinical situation explained to them and their family and to reassure them on what treatment options are available and what investigations might be required. If, early on in a clinic, a patient needs forty or fifty minutes to do this appropriately then the clinic is likely to run late. This is not often a problem if there are good staff managing the patient flow and explaining the situation to the patients who are waiting.

On the wards continuity of care is essential. It makes a huge difference to be able to go on to a ward to see a specific patient and know that you can find a nurse who knows the patient's case and who knows their recent observations and problems, this is becoming increasingly difficult. The management seem to have no real insight into the importance of this type of relationship, or if they do realise, they fear it might threaten their control.

For a surgeon, the area of his working day which is most dependent upon teamwork is probably the operating theatre environment. Again, I was extraordinarily fortunate to work with four or five anaesthetists whom I knew well and for whom I had an extremely high regard, in terms of their competence and care and their commitment to getting the job done irrespective of how long it might take. I also, almost always, had a theatre team whom I knew and who knew me. More recently management policies have deliberately tried to block the formation of theatre teams. Throughout an operation attention generally tends to be focussed on the surgeon and his assistants but in fact, usually, the most important person in the operating theatre is the anaesthetist.

It has always struck me as slightly ironical that patients seeking private surgery do not go to an anaesthetist first and say, "I trust you to keep me alive, so I will trust you to choose a surgeon for me". In many ways it would make more sense but that is just not the way it happens.

A good rapport between a surgeon and an anaesthetist, working in a familiar environment, is probably the single most important thing for patient safety and efficient use of operating theatre time.

When a new consultant job is created or an established post is to be replaced, a management team will draw up what is called a job description, which is really just a working programme on a weekly or monthly basis for the new appointee.

Considering the appointment of consultant anaesthetists, a job description traditionally would have involved a clear commitment to two or three surgeons. Anaesthetists, like other clinicians, have specialist fields of interest and expertise, so if a job is advertised for somebody with a strong background in, for instance, peripheral nerve blocks, one might expect their job description to involve developing a working commitment with surgeons operating most frequently on the limbs; this could be orthopaedic or plastic surgeons. The same sort of teamwork would apply for anaesthetists with a particular interest in children's anaesthesia, or operations involving the opening of the thoracic cavity; it is something around which a strong and effective team can be based.

This, of course, is considered a danger by the management and I know of Trusts where job descriptions for anaesthetists are now based upon no more than one or two fixed sessions a week. This means that at least three quarters of their work schedule will be changed from week to week, so they never know to which surgeon and where they will be allocated more than a week or two in advance. In a large hospital Trust employing perhaps 150 consultant anaesthetists, as well as many fellows and junior trainees, operating in a large number of different operating theatres on more than one site, it is probable that anaesthetists will be sent to do a list in a hospital they are not particularly familiar with, with a surgeon they have never seen before.

The scene is set for a situation where the following events could, or perhaps did, take place.

Each operating list starts with a meeting at which the surgical and anaesthetic teams introduce each other. This time-consuming ritual is only necessary because of the breakdown of team working patterns. The cases on the list are each discussed in terms of the surgical and anaesthetic input and the order and, for limb surgery, the side are confirmed. This absurdity is simply a manifestation of where adherence to protocols stops individuals from thinking in their own right. It does not mean that the order of the list doesn't change and doesn't stop the wrong limb being anaesthetised by a peripheral block (not infrequently, and with no serious long-term consequences) or rarely but still happening, the wrong side gets operated on.

An experienced and very senior anaesthetist was sent to a gynaecology operating list in a theatre he had never worked in before. He knew no one in the team, from surgeon to theatre orderly, and no one knew him. The first patient on the list was grossly obese, which is a good reason to avoid general anaesthesia, if possible, so the anaesthetist (who has a sense of humour) says that he will do the case under a spinal anaesthetic as anaesthesia is only required from the waist down and the patient can be comfortably sedated. The anaesthetic assistant says to the anaesthetist, "We haven't met before, where to you normally work?", and he replies, "well actually I am not really an anaesthetist, I am a vet". He goes on to explain that the management are so short of anaesthetists, which is true, that they are willing to persuade anybody who could give an anaesthetic to come and do a list, which is also true (more of this later). The anaesthetic assistant looks a little surprised but accepts the story and says "well this first patient could be exceedingly difficult for a spinal because they are grossly overweight. Where do you normally work?" The anaesthetist replies "I do quite a lot of work in Whipsnade Zoo. I know this first patient is very fat but I am quite used to doing spinal anaesthetics on elephants and rhinoceroses so I think if I can do it for a pachyderm, I should be able to do it for somebody with much thinner skin".

The case proceeds and goes well and the patient is returned to Recovery. The charade continues throughout the list with occasional asides from the anaesthetist such as, following a general anaesthetic, "well that seemed to go okay, time to wake her up and take her back to her owner, I mean return her to Recovery".

At the end of the list, in which there are, of course, no anaesthetic problems the anaesthetic assistant says goodbye, goes straight to a computer and fills in an online Datix complaint saying that they have just had to do a list with a vet. Fortunately, the Datix arrived on the computer of the next person up the management line, to whom the anaesthetist was well known, the matter went no further. If it had fallen into the management disciplinary mill there could have been quite silly consequences. It illustrates some important points.

The anaesthetic assistant's main concern was, as indoctrinated by management, that political correctness is more important than clinical safety. The frequently repeated management mantra that "patient wellbeing and safety is our prime concern" is simply a lie. Their prime concern is meeting targets and they are penalised for cancelling operating lists. The assistant had been instilled with the belief that cancelling a list is a crime which should be avoided at all costs, whereas political incorrectness is an even worse crime that must be allowed to run its full course and then rigorously punished. The management run mandatory training courses, the main purpose of which is to ensure the appropriate indoctrination of the clinical staff.

The managers have tried to replace teams, which they are afraid of, with Protocols, over which they have complete control, but, sadly, they seem to be ignorant of the difference between a routine and a protocol. The Oxford English Dictionary tells us that a routine is "a sequence of actions regularly followed" or "performed as part of a regular procedure". It is a pattern, acquired by the individual performing the procedure, to minimise the risk of omitting a vital part of the sequence. If there are several individuals involved in the procedure, who are all familiar with the routine (a team), then the risk of something being done wrong or forgotten becomes exceedingly small. A protocol is "the official system of rules governing affairs of state or diplomatic occasions" or "the accepted code of behaviour in a particular situation". To put it another way, how to behave when you are being introduced to a head of state. Not something that many of us have made a habit of being involved in or perform as part of a regular procedure. Not a pattern of behaviour acquired over many repetitions of an important procedure, thereby minimising the risk of a dangerous omission.

Protocols are a perfect management tool because they can be written by a management committee who have never in their lives performed the procedure in question and they do not even have to make any sense; but they can be used to justify their mantra of "patient safety first" in the event of almost any clinical mishap.

The Bard of Avon might have summarised it elegantly, if Twelfth Night was a comedy about the NHS, by explaining that "No one is born with a routine, some achieve routines, safely and usefully, but in The NHS the clinicians have Protocols thrust upon them".

Rare and potentially damaging events occur because a series of unlikely mistakes are made sequentially. This has been called the "Emmental cheese theory", which likens human systems to multiple slices of the Swiss cheese stacked on top of each other. Each slice has several holes in it and the risk of a problem occurring is compared to the chance of one hole in each slice lying immediately below and above a hole in the slice lying on each side of it. The greater the number of slices the less is the chance of something falling straight through the cheese.

I prefer the golfing analogy; the total space occupied by a tree is 80% air, but there is virtually no chance of successfully hitting a golf ball through the middle of the tree and the bigger the tree the less the chance. Applying this theory to a group of people involved in the management of a clinical case, any one of them might make a mistake but unless they all make the same mistake, sequentially, for different reasons, nothing untoward will happen. I will describe another clinical scenario.

An elderly lady is brought into an A&E Department by ambulance having sustained a fracture of her left hip at home. She is a little disorientated and is known to suffer from relatively mild senile dementia. She is seen by a casualty officer and an X-ray revealed that she had an unstable fracture of the proximal femur involving the hip joint and therefore technically called a fracture of the hip. This is best treated by surgery to fix the fracture and she is admitted to a Trauma Ward where she is "clerked in" (interviewed and examined) by another junior doctor. They start the necessary blood tests and paperwork preparatory to an operation but do not have time to complete all these things before their shift ended and her care is taken over by the next person coming on to work on the rota. They were aware that all the preparation for an operation has not been completed but that the patient has been examined. Without examining the patient themselves (it has already been done and there are a great many other patients requiring attention) they conclude the paperwork including getting the consent form signed; but the patient, by now thoroughly disorientated, says it is her right hip which is injured so that is the side consented for operation and marked with indelible ink.

The X-rays are not available on the ward as they are up on the X-ray viewing screens in the A&E Department for review and management discussion the following morning by the entire Trauma Team including consultants.

Those X-rays had been put up on the viewing screen back to front so that the left hip appeared on the right side.

The following morning the on-call consultant and his team hand over duty to a new consultant and team at a meeting held every morning to review all the X-rays of patients admitted in the previous 24-hours. These include the elderly lady with the fractured hip but by this time there is nobody at that meeting who had, physically, examined the *patient. That type of fracture of the hip joint leaves the injured leg short with the foot pointing outwards; it is a very characteristic deformity and anybody with the most rudimentary experience of trauma surgery would be able to recognise immediately which was the injured side.*

There is still a lot of tree for the golf ball to get through.

A surgical registrar is somebody who has been accepted on a training programme to become a specialist surgeon, in this case a Trauma and Orthopaedic Surgeon. This is considered a single specialty although the two aspects are a little different and people these days tend to specialise in one or the other. In multiple traumas, such as a severe road traffic accident, several specialists might be involved usually with one, probably the traumatologist, taking over-all supervisory control. For instance, a rupture of the great artery leaving the heart (the aorta) would require a thoracic surgeon (this, incidentally, is the injury which so tragically killed Princess Diana). A fractured pelvis and broken limbs would require the orthopaedic traumatologist, visceral damage in the abdomen such as a ruptured spleen would require an abdominal surgeon, a damaged liver would ideally be managed by a hepatobiliary surgeon and damage to the kidneys or bladder would be managed by a urologist. In a "simple" hip fracture only a trauma surgeon would be required.

For our elderly lady with the fractured left hip the team coming on duty for the subsequent 24-hours included, as the registrar on duty to perform the surgery, a trainee who had done quite a lot of orthopaedics but has just moved that day to the Trauma Department, which might be effectively completely separate from, or even in a separate hospital from, the Orthopaedic Department. Although considered a competent technical surgeon for his level of experience he has done no fracture fixation. A second registrar, who has been training on the Trauma Service for many months and is experienced in the fixation of fractures is available that morning with no other specific commitment and it is arranged that the two of them should operate together to fix the patient's fracture, although the belief is that it is a fracture of right hip because of the misplacement of the X-rays.

The registrar new to trauma and the experienced trauma registrar are both somewhat arrogant, but otherwise of differing personalities and temperaments and rather dislike each other. The new one resents being told to take over the management of a patient who had not been admitted under his care and the other one resents being made to hang around to supervise someone who is not really capable of doing the operation on their own. Neither of them goes to see the patient before going to the operating theatre as neither of them feel any particular personal responsibility for the patient, who has been discussed at the morning meeting in the usual way. They probably both have other things that need their attention and they probably do not hurry to the operating theatre as early as they should.

Meanwhile the anaesthetist and the anaesthetic assistant have assembled in theatre and the theatre nursing team are ready, so the patient is sent for from the ward. On the ward everyone is busy at the start of the morning, but she is checked out with all the necessary paperwork and the porters take her to the theatres on her bed. The patient and her paperwork are checked in by theatre reception and handed over to the care of the anaesthetic nurse and the anaesthetist in the specific theatre expecting her. They check the paperwork and check that the side consented for operation is the side marked and administer a general anaesthetic with the patient still in the bed, because moving her would be very painful.

Once all the monitoring and intravenous access is in place the patient is moved from the anaesthetic room into the operating theatre. For fixing this type of hip fracture the patient is put on a special table with the foot on the fractured side strapped into a boot which enables traction to be applied to the limb in order to help re-orientate (reduce) the fracture to a more anatomical position. This is undertaken by the theatre orderlies, the X-ray is placed on a screen, but everyone is expecting an operation on the right side and 2 views of the fractured left hip are again put up back to front to assist with the surgery, but not leaving enough room to display the right (unfractured) hip. Everything is set up for the right (incorrect) hip to be operated on.

The ball still has a long way to go to emerge from the tree.

Once the patient is positioned on the table an X-ray imaging device is moved in to take an X-ray of the hip to be operated on and this is displayed on a monitor screen. Of course, it shows a hip with no fracture, but the traction had already been applied and the X-ray is correctly displayed on the screen giving the impression that the fractured hip is the *one now being displayed by the current X-ray device on the monitor.*

The patient is now ready to be prepared for surgery and the surgeons arrive. Probably they look at the consent form, they look at the X-ray, and they look at the recent image of the hip at the present time on the table displayed on the monitor. Their main interest is to check that the X ray imager is in the correct place to show the bones as they insert the metal fixation device. They come to the very strange conclusion that the traction alone has produced an anatomical reduction of the fracture so that it is not visible on the X-ray monitor screen. This is absolutely not possible for this type of unstable fracture. I imagine that the surgeon with an experience of fractures did not really check the supposed reduction and the one with no fracture experience did not know any better. The surgery commences and again, I imagine that the surgeon with fracture experience does not scrub to take part in the operation but merely remains present to show how the instrumentation should be used. The bone is exposed but on incising the soft tissues, if there is a fracture present, there would be quite extensive bruising between the skin and the bone. This cannot have been present in an unfractured hip, but nobody remarks on this. The bolt and plate held by screws are inserted under vision using the X-ray machine. It is not difficult to insert a fracture fixation device into a bone that has no fracture and I imagine that a satisfactory position of the metalwork is achieved and confirmed with the X-ray monitor. The wound is closed, the patient is returned to recovery and then to the ward and a check X-ray is taken and placed on the screens in the Trauma

Department to be reviewed by the team finishing their on-call and the team taking over the next morning.

At that meeting the next morning it is finally recognised that the bolt and screws have been inserted in the unfractured hip and the fractured side has not been operated on at all. The golf ball has emerged from the leafy tree on its original trajectory.

Such a fluke shot in golf would be talked about for 100 years.

The patient returns to theatre the following day and the correct hip is fixed by a senior fellow. The frail patient does not survive two operations within 48 hours.

If you think that this could not happen, think again. If you think that it should not happen, you are absolutely right. So how does this sort of thing happen? The explanation of course is that all the holes in the cheese had formed in alignment which is a several thousand to one shot.

Going through the sequence of events there are at least 25 people or occasions when one or more individual could have spotted that a grave error had been made and was being perpetuated.

All the protocols have been followed but two mistakes have not been picked up, the consent and the original orientation of the X ray. All the protocols and checks and cross-checks and boxes ticked that any manager can ever dream up will not absolutely prevent this from happening. This is termed a "never event" meaning that it should never happen, but of course never events do happen which makes it a fundamentally silly name. The management response to this situation would be to introduce more protocols, more boxes to tick, more forms to fill in, which will only make this situation even worse and the error more likely to occur again. The clinicians have been deliberately conditioned to stop thinking and just respond to structured patterns of work and exchange of information.

The only things that will reduce the risk of something like this happening, if not to never, then at least to the level where it is an event that is talked about for a hundred years, are two concepts which are central to the successful undertaking of any endeavour, ranging from warfare to sport and including things like teaching, diplomacy, and healthcare delivery.

These two things are continuity of care/responsibility/interest; and teamwork. In medicine continuity of care/responsibility should be maintained at least for any given in-patient episode. It may not be realistic to continue it beyond that, but interest, at least, could be maintained. Continuity has been made difficult by the politicians as I will mention in the next chapter, but teamwork has been deliberately suppressed by the managerial staff employed by the NHS, which I think is probably an Orwellian plot in their attempts to intimidate, dominate and thus control the clinicians. It is part of why they love shifting people around within the workplace. Only by working with people that one admires, respects and trusts can an individual care about the performance of others within their team. The team worker does not want their friends and colleagues to perform poorly. They do not want mistakes made by the group they identify with and that group remains, to paraphrase recent political slogans, "alert and keen to control the risk and protect the NHS", on behalf of the entire team.

So, the managers find themselves in a position where their ability to perform well is judged very largely on their ability to control clinicians. They do this by minimising the clinician's ability to work with each other by forming teams, and by trying to impose hard outcomes as a measure of performance. Managers love protocols but their value in clinical care is extremely limited at best and can be actively harmful at worst. Many management dictates are therefore actually damaging to the delivery of healthcare and their response to every new problem is to proliferate and create a new tier of themselves.

They use the blame culture they have created to intimidate the clinicians into accepting responsibility for unfortunate, but unforeseeable events; things like rare intra-operative complications, falls on a ward when a confused patient goes for a wander in the middle of the night, previously unknown allergic reactions to drugs, the list is a long one. These risks in general should have been, and usually will have been discussed with and understood by the patient and their family from the outset. But increasingly the clinician is instructed to write a letter of apology to the patient's family if any such thing occurs. This can, I think, be misconstrued as an admission of some sort of guilt, which is probably very unfair on the clinician and which creates a doubt and dilemma in the minds of the relatives. A chance, perhaps, of increasing the staff in the management's complaints department?

I started this chapter by saying that most of the managers I have personally had dealings with are pleasant, well-motivated and well-intentioned individuals. Although I have gone on to attempt to explain why I believe they are a very large part of why the whole system is failing, that initial observation remains my fundamental belief; but with the very clear exception of one particular group of managers. This is both a personal observation and a generalisation so it should not be thought of out of the context of the limitations that those two assessments carry.

It is my experience that the most ineffective and, above all, vindictive group of NHS managers are those who were clinicians but have, relatively late in their career, changed to being pure managers and strategists. This is another of the paradoxes which I find myself acknowledging. One would think that a clinician would have the best insight into how healthcare should be delivered and indeed that should be the case and sometimes is, but the vast majority seem to me to be bitter and disillusioned. I have a theory as to why this should be.

Most students who train in Medicine do so with the belief that it will lead, ultimately to treating patients, but Medicine, perhaps more than any other career, is immensely diverse. As people pass through their undergraduate and postgraduate training, they find a huge variety of fields in which they might choose to pursue a career. Although most people end up dealing with patients in one form or another, some end up in pure basic science research and never see a patient and others end up in clinical fields like pathology where patient contact is rare or non-existent. Some find that they enjoy direct contact with patients and others find it difficult. Medicine can accommodate all these widely differing ambitions and desires, but I think very few people start, or even finish, their postgraduate training with the specific intention of going into NHS Management.

There are many sayings in clinical medicine which, as with other fields of life, are often half in jest but also represent at least a half truth. For instance, in terms of acquiring the skill for a particular procedure "see one, do one, teach one". In terms of describing, for a relatively rare clinical problem, one's experience and expertise "I have some experience of this" means I have seen it once and "I have seen this again and again" means I have seen this twice, whilst "I have seen this time after time after time" means I have seen this on at least three occasions. There is also a saying that "if you can't do it, teach it". It is certainly the case that most individuals who are good at something within their profession get their professional satisfaction out of doing it and those that are not particularly good at doing something become frustrated.

My impression is that people who have the title of Professor are usually better at talking about something than they are at doing it, but I believe that the "if you can't" path goes beyond teaching. The next stage is "if you can't teach it, examine in it". A frustrated clinician could try becoming a teacher and might be very good at it, but if their communication skills are poor, the next stage would be to try examining in the subject. By this time, they may be becoming bitter, which produces the worst type of examiner.

A good examiner realises that their main role is to give the candidate the best possible opportunity of showing their knowledge and passing the exam, but an angry examiner believes that their role is really to try and frustrate and trick the candidate and, if at all possible, to fail them. I have seen both types of examiners but, in this new age of enlightenment, an examiner who fails an excessively high proportion of candidates will, eventually, be weeded out and stopped from examining. The last professional option open to them, given that they can't examine in a subject, is to manage it; by which time they have a deep-seated dislike of the career system and an intensely vindictive attitude towards those people who can do the clinical things that they could not.

It is a personal opinion. Whether there is any truth in it or not, I neither know nor care, but going into management is certainly a very lucrative and easy way to pass the last ten years or so of one's career whilst working towards a satisfactory pension. I will discuss how this sad pathway could be changed in the next chapter.

Chapter 4

Politicians and the NHS: an unnecessarily uneasy relationship?

It is certainly true that no private corporation or charity would have both the motivation and the power to create a state healthcare delivery system, therefore we must acknowledge our gratitude to politicians for the creation of the National Health Service in the first place. Although Bevan had to work hard to persuade the medical profession, partly represented by an intransigent BMA, to accept it in 1947 it is probably the case that by the early 1950s most clinicians in this country had reached a point where they found themselves in agreement with the concept of a nationalised health service. They felt that in general it was no worse than what preceded it, in some respects it was a vast improvement, providing a reasonably pleasant environment in which they could concentrate on their clinical role within the community.

Perhaps the politicians were so incensed by the BMA's attitude in 1947 and 8 that they developed a profound aversion to all clinicians which has been passed on, like an inherited disease, to successive governments ever since. Maybe the doctors, who can be somewhat arrogant and over-bearing (possibly more so in the early years of the NHS than now) have similarly acquired and passed on over the years a resentment of any structure being imposed upon them. Whatever the origin they now deeply dislike and distrust one another. There continues to be some justification for a little wariness from both groups, but that really needs to be resolved. They should both be pulling in the same direction, together, as a team; after all they both want the same outcome – a strong, successful, efficient and cost-effective health care delivery system. Any of them who do not should resign and move on.

I am, by nature, somebody who believes in the maximum of free enterprise and the minimum of state intervention. I do not really like the idea of nationalised industries, however there are some things that I think clearly need to be run as a nationalised enterprise; the military for instance and, I believe, health care delivery systems.

Privatisation is not always a good thing. It does not seem that the railways are very well run as a group of private corporations, although the national road network is not a lot better. Piecemeal privatisation is probably the worst of both worlds.

I believe passionately in the National Health Service and I believe that it should be enlarged and extended. None of it should be privatised, but I think there needs to be some local flexibility in management strategies, once again, one size does not fit all.

I have tried to review the input of successive politicians to the NHS over the years, but it struck me as the mental equivalent of trying to untangle a large bowl of spaghetti using only a toothpick held in your non-dominant hand. It constitutes a large volume of verbiage and is neither appropriate nor necessary for this small work.

There are, however, some clear patterns that emerge which explain, perhaps, some of the continuing antipathy between politicians and clinicians that needs to be resolved.

All politicians recognise that, despite the "national disgrace" group, the NHS is dear to the heart of most of the electorate. They should be dissuaded from making extravagant and unrealistic promises about health care delivery in their attempts to secure votes.

No one political party or doctrine has provided the majority of bad, or good, structural changes. These are all presented in meaningless newspeak political jargon like "Change for Good", "Choose and Book", "Internal Market" or "Integrated Care", but it matters not one iota which government created them.

All Shadow Ministers of Health are vehemently opposed to any government minister's health care reforms and scrap them the moment they come into power. If they do. They usually then re-introduce them under another name within one or two years of being in government.

Whether the changes in themselves are good or bad, popular or unpopular or from the left or right wing of the political spectrum is irrelevant. The damage to continuity and morale is wrought by their sheer number and frequency.

The BMA invariably objects to everything.

Having said that it is their number, rather than their nature, which is so destructive I would like to give a few examples of political edicts which have been a source of personal annoyance for me over the last thirty years. I will try to attribute them where possible. The first two have been imposed on us by the EU, but I suppose we may now have disentangled ourselves from that.

Politicians gave us The European Working Time Directive. This is an EU law passed in 1998, but because of the profound effect it had on the working patterns of junior doctors it was gradually phased in and did not become fully effective in the NHS until August 2009. It was intended to protect people generally from inhumane working hours and conditions, for doctors its justification was that they should not be expected to work when they were tired, which was considered dangerous. As often seems to happen with EU laws the road of good intentions went over a cliff.

It is a complicated bill with many clauses and a theoretical option for individuals to withdraw from it but, in essence, it forced the permitted hours of work per week down from 56 to 48, averaged over six months. Worse than that, job plans had to be constructed so that people only worked an average of 8 hours per 24 and everyone had 11 hours of consecutive rest per day. Being resident on call at night counts as work, even if there is nothing to do, so a night possibly spent sleeping MUST be followed by a day off. The complexities of allowing any individual to opt out of these restrictions are unmanageable for a junior doctor trainee work force which rotates every 2,3,4 or 6 months, so some employing trusts simplified things by saying that any time spent at work outside the EU law would not be indemnified against legal action.

All of this has done a great deal of damage to junior doctor's training and, more importantly, to continuity of patient care in hospitals. Most junior doctors are very keen to spend as much time as possible watching and learning from clinical situations, especially to follow the outcomes for a patient whose management plan they have been involved in formulating.

Politicians also gave us European Employment Law, a collection of binding regulations intended to protect workers' rights across the EU, introduced over many years and constantly being updated.

Regarding the NHS, it states that EU citizens applying for a clinical post, such as a one-year fellowship must, by law, be selected over a non-EU applicant, provided they have comparable (very vague) qualifications. Furthermore, it is against the law to discriminate against any EU citizen based on language skills. These two legal stipulations may, of course, be mutually exclusive. Whatever a doctor's qualifications and experience are in their home nation they cannot fulfil a clinical role for a nation in whose language they are unable to communicate. I had a permanent headache for the first three months of my year in France, but I was working in a clinical research role, not making clinical management decisions. By the end of the year, I was dreaming in French, but I would still have struggled with a busy clinic.

The resolution decided between The Home Office and the GMC, was that EU Law takes precedence; thus, after generations of making a vital contribution to the functioning of the NHS, subjects of The Commonwealth (India, Canada, Africa and Australasia had all sent many particularly outstanding young doctors and nurses) could not be appointed if there was an EU applicant, who could not be language tested, whereas all other applicants would have to pass a language test.

I had one applicant whom I was particularly keen to appoint as he was highly recommended by several Australian colleagues and friends who had been contemporaries of mine in training. He was a Greek Australian who had dual nationality, but all his education and training had been in Australia. His Greek citizenship meant that he could get a Work Permit, but The GMC decided that his Australian nationality and training meant that he had to sit the language test. No problem, he sat it. He failed, so he sat it again. He failed a second time, but this time he felt it could not just be a clerical error and made enquiries. He was told that no one with a Greek name like his and a work permit granted because of Greek nationality could be expected to achieve such a high score, so he must have cheated by getting someone else to sit the test for him. He sat it a third time with an invigilator, but I do not think he was refunded two of the three fees he had paid to register for the test.

Perhaps, now, this kind of nonsense will cease.

However poor the clinicians may be at structure and organisation it seems to me that the people best able to decide what services should be provided by a health care delivery system are the clinicians themselves. They are in the position to make an informed and disinterested decision as to what constitutes a worthwhile clinical intervention and what priority, if any, it should be given. The politicians are always at risk of being unduly influenced by vocal, passionate and emotive campaigns instigated by pressure groups who may influence voting patterns.

For instance, should it be the state's responsibility to provide In Vitro Fertilisation (IVF) services free at the point of delivery? I do not know the answer, it is not my field of expertise. The only people who can answer that question and to whose judgement I would happily bow, are those clinicians who provide that service. Joint replacement was my field, it has always been my very strongly held opinion that it is NOT the state's responsibility to provide a "prompt", free at the point of delivery hip replacement for an 80-year-old man who owns and lives in a £2.5 million house and has a large index linked pension, just to enable him to play golf at his local exclusive club. If such a patient genuinely believes that it is the state's responsibility to provide him with a "lifestyle" hip replacement, then that is what should be done, but the timely fashion would be a long wait on clinical grounds. His treatment is nowhere near as urgent as that of an elderly man living alone in a council flat who is awake all night with intractable pain and who is struggling to maintain his independence. I will return to this example later in this chapter.

There are endless examples of these paradoxes which I used to enjoy putting to the medical students. Should the state, for instance, refuse to provide services to drug addicts, including people who drink more than the recommended levels of alcohol per week or who smoke tobacco in some form? Should the state provide healthcare to people who are morbidly obese? These are easy questions to answer, of course the NHS is obliged to take all comers, including "high risk" patients. Not so easy is the question of whether the state should provide a eugenics service for abortion of pregnancies where the mother wants a son, not a daughter, or vice versa. This of course should never really occur, but it is not difficult for the mother to claim that she is too mentally unstable to face continuing with the pregnancy and would pose a risk to the wellbeing of the child if it were not terminated.

Should the state provide cosmetic surgical services? Generally, the students would say no to this before they began to think about the sixteen-year-old girl who has breast asymmetry with failure of development on one side, or the sixty-year-old woman whose breasts have become so pendulous that she has to fasten her skirt over them at the level of her waist. When does cosmetic surgery in the hands of a plastic surgeon become reconstructive surgery? There should be some element of cosmesis in all forms of surgery. Should the state provide a service for the removal of tattoos? That usually got them. There would be howls of "no, under no circumstances" until it was suggested that they consider the victims of branding in concentration camps who just want to get rid of, for instance, the Auschwitz number tattooed onto their wrists. These are all dilemmas that can only be resolved by clinicians on an individual basis. Attempts by politicians or, at one remove, the health care purchasing authorities to provide "one rule fits all" solutions are doomed to painful failure. Painful, that is, to those patients who believe they have fallen on the wrong side of the rule, and they may be right in believing that.

There must be some financial control over what is offered as an NHS service, but the clinicians should lead it. This will not be easy to monitor but, given that dilemmas only really arise over elective services, there is time for consideration. Perhaps individual applications could be made by clinicians, on behalf of patients, to a review body. It sounds a bit cumbersome, like planning permission for buildings, but one rule does not fit all.

The politicians play a despicable role in creating false expectations in the minds of the general public. This fosters the incredibly difficult to manage "I know my rights" aggressive behaviour on the part of the public, particularly in high pressure areas like Accident and Emergency Departments. The simplest example of this is the endless pre-election promises of how many tens of thousands of new nurses and doctors are going to be recruited following an election victory by either party. This is so palpably a nonsense that I do not know why any politician even tries it, let alone expects it to be believed. Maybe politicians just have a very low opinion of the public's intelligence.

It takes three years for a nurse to qualify and at least another two years for them to become confident and experienced. It takes at least four years and usually five or even six years for a doctor to qualify and at least another six years for them to complete their postgraduate training. This of course easily outlasts the maximum term that any government can serve without calling a further election.

But by far the worst example of political interference was from Blair's huge majority government in the late 1990's. The infamous imposition of mandatory performance targets, both in terms of clinical turnover and financial management. One of the consequences of new rules about what must or must not be done is that there needs to be some form of control and retribution when the legal obligation is not undertaken or fulfilled. Government regulations and restrictions imposed as an attempt to control the coronavirus pandemic are a classic example of this. Some people, including members of, or advisors to, the government itself did not understand them, or agree with them and know they can ignore them with impunity because they are effectively un-enforceable, so there will be no meaningful retribution. A Rule or Law should never be imposed without first identifying the means for detecting disobedience and subsequently punishing it.

It is said, anecdotally, that these targets were the result of a casual conversation in which Blair asked how long people had to wait for elective surgery in the National Health Service and was told it was about eighteen months. His response was to say, "that's unacceptable. It should be eighteen weeks" and instantly an eighteen-week target was imposed. The idea of a maximum four hour wait in an A&E Department was similarly arbitrarily decided on.

The problem then was how to enforce it or punish the providers if it is not met. The political solution to that was to fine the relevant department of the healthcare delivery service. When an organisation is told to do something that is inevitably going to have increased expenditure consequences, then punished, when they fail to meet the demand, by reducing their budget is nonsensical in the extreme; but this is precisely what happens.

But it is not the logistical stupidity of the targets which is most galling, it is the fact that, once again, this kind of one rule fits all belief is simply not applicable to healthcare delivery. In an Accident and Emergency Department, for instance, patients are assessed, usually by a specialist nurse, on arrival, for the potential severity of their injury or presenting complaint. This is known as clinical triage and, if properly applied, is an effective way of ensuring that those with a life or limb threatening problem are treated most urgently. Even the most aggressive "I know my rights" merchant might feel a little embarrassed if he had his cut finger dressed because he had been waiting for 3 hours 55 minutes while someone else who had only come in 10 minutes ago bled to death on a trolley.

A&E Departments were noticeably quiet during the pandemic lockdown. There are likely to be many reasons for this, some more significant than others, but I suspect that one of them is that, usually, many patients attending for advice have no real need to be there at all and the risk of Covid infection changed their thinking.

Regarding elective surgery (that is "quality of life" procedures for generally not life or limb threatening conditions) time scale targets are a particularly crude and mindless bludgeon with which to, supposedly, improve provider performance. In the example I have given earlier of the two men seeking a hip replacement, one with pain only when playing golf and the other in constant inescapable pain, their differing financial circumstances are irrelevant. Clinically the one in constant pain should always take some degree of priority, by just how many days, weeks or months is a judgement that only the clinician in charge of their care can make. They may not always get it right, there could be a thousand variables to consider, but they should at least have the freedom to make the best and most equitable judgement they can.

I only threw in the affluence factor because it is a specific circumstance that I have encountered on numerous occasions and because the man who wants a prompt treatment to play golf might well, if given the right incentive, be happy to make some contribution towards the cost. There should be a mechanism for that to be possible, even perhaps encouraged. I suggest such a mechanism in chapter 11.

Targets on a timescale alone are pointless and damaging, leading to a grossly unfair system of health care delivery, but it takes a non-clinical vote seeking politician to fail to realise this.

A target on a numbers basis is a different matter, which certainly can be beneficial to patients if managed properly. This was not the result of a direct political edict, but probably came about as a result of Thatcher's NHS and Community Care Act of 1990 which created what was known as The Internal Market. It separated the role of The Purchasing Authority from The Provider of Care enabling hospitals to become semi-autonomous NHS Trusts. It was, of course, greeted with much scepticism from some doctors and point-blank obstruction from the BMA who saw it as the first step on the road to privatisation (having, in 1946, so stridently objected to nationalisation). In fact, it admirably focused the minds of the purchasers as to just what service they were buying and of the providers as to how they should provide the care to ensure that it was purchased from them in the future.

When I started my postgraduate surgical training programme the list of patients waiting for elective surgery was effectively the property of each individual consultant surgeon. It represented those patients that the consultant or his junior team had seen in an outpatient clinic and listed for a planned operation. Each week operating schedules were organised for a week or two following and it was one of the responsibilities of the junior trainees to choose what procedures should be done. The consequence of this was, not surprisingly, that those operations which were unusual or particularly interesting, or particularly likely to come up as part of an examination, would be chosen ahead of those operations which were considered "mundane". The result, inevitably, was a very inequitable waiting time for different surgical procedures and very short notice for the unsuspecting patients to make all the arrangements to be admitted to hospital for an operation.

It would also have been considered an unacceptable breech of etiquette for one consultant to take over the care of another consultant's patient, as listed, without specifically being requested to do so. This led to what I described, at the time (although not to any consultant himself) as penis envy (virtually all surgeons in those days were men). A sort of boastful, "my waiting list is bigger than your waiting list" culture. It was also, I am sad to say, used by consultants as an anvil on which to hammer patients into going privately; "I am afraid my waiting time for that procedure is at least three years, but I could do you privately next week". Some consultants also encouraged their juniors and secretarial staff to use this persuasive ploy on their behalf.

Let me give an example. Surgeon A has a five-year waiting time for an elective surgical procedure for bunions (a degenerative deformity of the big toe causing a painful bony protuberance) called a Keller's arthroplasty. This is a relatively simple but somewhat destructive procedure (was done very frequently, now quite rare) first described by W L Keller (a US Army Surgeon) in 1904. In the 1980s, foot surgery was not really a sub-specialty in orthopaedics and most orthopaedic surgeons dabbled in it with a greater or lesser degree of interest and expertise. In general, a Keller's procedure would always be undertaken by a trainee surgeon and virtually never by the consultant himself on an NHS list. In the same hospital, Surgeon B was charged with responsibility for the surgical training programme and had many surgical trainees attached to his service. Consequently, his waiting time for a Keller's arthroplasty was five months.

Given the unpredictable clinical outcomes following this procedure there is no way that Surgeon A could claim to offer a twelve times better chance of a good result than Surgeon B. This is particularly so given that for both the consultant surgeons the operation would almost certainly be undertaken by one of the trainees on their service. Whilst you might know the quality and experience of the trainees that were going to be with you in five months' time, there would have been no way that you could have known that five years in advance. But, of course, there was no question of some of the patients from Surgeon A being transferred to the care of Surgeon B thereby diminishing the size of Surgeon A's penis, I mean waiting list.

In 1987, I was appointed as a Consultant Orthopaedic Surgeon to work solely in the field of hip and knee arthritis and revision surgery. That is, mainly, hip and knee replacements. It was a newly created post and so I "inherited" no waiting list. Only three of my nine established senior consultant colleagues asked me to take over the care of some of their patients whom they felt were in dire clinical need of a joint replacement as quickly as possible.

Happily, the "internal market" empowered the management to break this malign practice.

That is the best thing that I have seen come out of management in forty years.

The lists became the property of the providing service or hospital and management assumed the role, with variable success, of spreading them equitably in terms of waiting time. Initially some patients were quite reluctant to "change their consultant in mid-stream". But they quickly realised the benefit of having been given a provisional date for surgery and have now become accustomed to the concept that they have been referred to a service rather than to an individual. I have no problem with an operation being performed by a surgeon who did not originally list the patient for the procedure, provided the operating surgeon discusses things with the patient beforehand and takes the formal Patient Consent. I do believe that the operating surgeon should then continue those patients care for as long as is necessary, if possible. Continuity of care is important, as I have said earlier, but just how important must be an individual clinician judgement.

All a good thing for patients, but then the waiting time targets were introduced and that has made it very difficult for any consultant to put together a planned operating list based on his judgement of clinical need. The overriding priority has become length of waiting time and it has now reached the point where surgeons can be disciplined for offering to operate on one patient ahead of their allocated time in the queue, irrespective of clinical priorities. That is a bad thing.

There is one final problem with which the population of many nations are burdening, to an increasingly dangerous extent, their health care delivery systems. Obesity. The Covid-19 infection was quickly declared a pandemic but, in the first wave at least, it was not an epidemic in the UK (it is the difference between geographical extent and localised incidence). We are now suffering a major and increasing obesity epidemic. We are one of the worst affected countries in the world and the responsibility for this lies, very largely, with successive governments of varying political inclinations. This could be the subject of an entire book, but I will restrict my observations to three examples of governments not acting responsibly in caring for the well-being of the people they were elected to serve. The most obvious is the unrestricted licencing and advertising of appalling fast/junk food outlets. Equally damaging, thinking of energy output rather than calorie consumption, was the mindless selling of school playing fields to property speculators for short term gain. These are both for commercial interests and likely to come from the right wing of political inclination.

Compounding this, from the aspect of both output and intake, is the perverted political perception that inequality is intrinsically evil, so any form of sport is bad for children because of its competitive nature; there will be winners and that may "damage" the losers. Inequality is part of life, as is not always having things go "your way", and the sooner children learn that the better. It is a consistent failing of the left wing of political inclination to confuse equality of opportunity, a particularly important good thing, with equality of outcome, an impossibility except by imposing restrictive injustice and thus a disastrously bad thing. So, they believe it is in children's "best interests" for them not to be offered and encouraged to take the opportunity to run around outside, but to sit at home eating junk food and living in the fantasy world of computer war games. Nobody loses, you just hit the replay button, get fat and die from the (very expensive) complications of type 2 diabetes.

It took a viral pandemic for politicians to realise how damaging obesity is to every aspect of good health and, incidentally, how important exercise is. Now they are going to throw more money at bariatric surgery, that is the technical term for partial, irreversible, surgical evisceration to reduce calorie absorption.

This is like a society blocking access to contraception but providing an abortion service. How twisted is that thinking? Have they not realised that prevention is infinitely better (and less dangerous and expensive) than cure?

So, overall, I think the influence of the various political factions (Parties?) has been pretty much neutral. Their bad influence stems from the fact that they all tend to be competitive animals and cannot resist changing anything that has been set up by their opponents, or promising greater benefits than any of their rivals.

The age of the "public servant" politician is gone forever, which is probably a good thing as it stemmed only from unbridled privilege or rabid fanaticism.

Our society is constantly evolving in terms of our expectations and aspirations, as is the provision of healthcare. To balance these two changing forces requires a strategy and a delivery system with far greater stability than the politics of a democracy, but certainly not with the bullying rigidity of a dictatorship.

Perhaps the perfect blend is unattainable. Politicians, despite their competitive urge for change, are the elected representatives of society and must be involved; ultimately, they hold the purse strings.

I believe there are two changes that might help.

The first would be to find some way of damping down the extravagant promises and the quick-fire changes that sequential governments are unable to resist. It would take a constitutional expert to envisage how this could be achieved, but could a group of distinguished public, or not so public, figures be created to impose a longer term stability on the political input. Perhaps a retired politician or two; people will have their own thoughts, mine, at the moment, would be John Major and Gordon Brown. Perhaps some successful philanthropists from commerce; in the past Viscount Nuffield would have been perfect. Some retired senior civil servants, some academics, some from the judiciary; perhaps, just now, a senior member of the Royal

Family, The Princess Royal, with The Duke of Cambridge in mind to succeed her?

The second would be to find a way of getting more, above all better, input from the clinicians. We should be looking at creating a situation where health care strategy and management are a prestigious and attractive career option for clinicians in a postgraduate training scheme. Perhaps a training programme could be created with various options for a clinical speciality which would be taken to the point of being able to run an independent clinical practice (call it consultant-level or associate specialist-level) but which would have as its main thrust the development and application of skills required for good management strategies from a clinical perspective. Could we even end up with a Royal College of Health Care Management?

Chapter 5
Litigation and the NHS

The regulation of any professional group is an exceedingly difficult balance, perhaps, not surprisingly, impossible to achieve perfectly. One cannot please all the people all of the time; if it was a mathematical model it would be something like, a number representing expertise in the field in question multiplied by a number for impartiality and divided by a number for judicial experience. The numbers are all a guess, so the resultant solution is infinitely variable. The difficulty applies to the police and the law, the military, the financial services, journalism, etc., only politics seems exempt.

But it is particularly emotive in the field of health care delivery. Every aspect of that field should be open to public scrutiny and performance evaluation; probably more so for private than public, the powerful incentive of profit margins cannot be ignored. Another reason why it is safest that it should all be public.

The regulation of the whole of health care delivery is too vast a topic to discuss in a single chapter and I do not propose to try. I will concern myself merely with the regulation of the medical profession, but the regulation of other clinical groups, such as nurses and therapists, is, I believe, basically similar.

In theory, for doctors, it should rest with The General Medical Council, overseeing peer review with the medical director of the employing trust, who should also respond to comments from The Care Quality Commission. But in practice the day-to-day governance of clinical activity does not; it rests, very largely, with the whim of the patients, in the hands of the legal profession.

Clinical Negligence is where a treatment has breached "the duty of care", resulting in an injury or illness. Once again, we are left trying to assess a soft outcome, or judgement; what is an acceptable, or, more pertinently, an unacceptable "duty of care". There is a general belief among clinicians that if five reputable practitioners, in the relevant field, agree that a treatment was reasonable within the concept of recognized professional standards (another soft judgement) then it does not breach the duty of care. As is so often the case in life, this is probably, at best, a compromise, but it is also seriously flawed. It would virtually always be possible to identify five practicing clinicians who would state that they have provided a similar duty of care on many occasions; but their clinical competence is not in question and perhaps it should be. Conversely, one so called "expert witness" with a particularly obsessional belief in a given treatment regime can obstinately and irreversibly refuse to accept that another option is reasonable.

This, in turn, raises the question of what precisely defines an "expert witness". A proportion of consultant clinicians are attracted to a medico-legal practice for various reasons. I think it appeals to a particular personality for whom reading, reflection and debate seem more rewarding than clinical action. As I have said before a career in medicine can match the widest and most catholic spread of aspirations imaginable.

But it is also another form of private practice, that is, work undertaken outside the hours of NHS contract, for remuneration over and above the NHS salary and, like clinical private practice, it is not really regulated in any satisfactory way. Medico-legal cases are often "added" to NHS clinics and the time spent thinking and writing about them is not specifically identified. Solicitors, not surprisingly, will tend to seek an opinion from someone they work with regularly and whom they can rely on to respond quickly. They, like estate agents selling a house, have more interest in the turn-around time than any degree of expertise for the specifics in question. Furthermore, a lot of doctors will carry on with a medico-legal practice long after they have retired from any clinical work. They simply cannot be familiar with current practice.

If the expertise of the medical experts is often in doubt so, alas, is the wisdom of many of the settlements arrived at by the lawyers (there is a statutory obligation for the claimant's and the defendant's teams to seek a "deal" before the matter is brought to court, if possible) or the judges if the case does come to court.

The Law is an extremely complicated beast which, like most things, is subject to the influence of ignorance and prejudice. Happily, I have little close experience or knowledge of negligence litigation, but, as an observer, it seems clear to me that outcomes are often reached, both by agreement and as a court ruling, by a fairly circuitous and mysterious route. One thing that does seem to have a considerable influence is consideration of prior judgements in similar cases. This can lead to a cascade of Chinese whispers, where the similarity between a case under review and the defining prior judgement of a case becomes more and more tenuous, but the prior judgement still decides the case.

Say, a new ruling is made in Case A, setting a precedent. Case B is similar to case A, so the prior ruling prevails. Case C is similar to Case B, which now constitutes the prior ruling; and so on until we get to Case N, which is similar to Case M, the current prior ruling, but is nothing like Case A. "The Law" has become "an ass"; the law is not always the same as justice.

An example of this was a Supreme Court judgement in 2015, the Montgomery ruling. It revolves around what constitutes informed consent from patients undergoing an operation and changed the legal test for determining what is sufficient disclosure. The legal weight was shifted from what a reasonable doctor would warn the patient about to what a reasonable patient would expect to know. Apparently, the Supreme Court believed that the ruling would reduce litigation, but, by the law of unintended consequences, it just blurred the requirements for what a patient should be told. It is now virtually impossible to defend an allegation by a patient that they were not properly informed before their operation. Payments for these allegations have soared from £25 million in 2011 to £62 million in 2019.

I do not believe any clinician would want to return to the days when so many patients would respond to information with a cheerful "Whatever you say Doctor, you know best." Not always true, quite apart from anything else. I recall a consultant surgeon's ward round (I was a clinical medical student hiding at the back of the "Sir Lancelot Spratt style entourage" and terrified of being asked a question) where the great man (his own estimate) was presented to a patient he was going to operate on the next day. He said something like "Good afternoon Madam, you have a small ulcer on the back passage. I am going to operate tomorrow and when you wake up the bowel will open on the side. Good day to you". This was to describe an irreversible partial evisceration requiring a colostomy; I like to think the "entourage" explained things a little better later.

Things are a lot better than that now, but the fact is that "informed consent" in the sense that the Montgomery ruling has come to be applied is a myth.

Patients who have been unlucky in ending up with an unusually bad outcome from a treatment might disagree, but it is a fact that a complication or disappointing result does not automatically equate to negligence in the selection or administration of a treatment program. Even when the patients were clearly warned of the possibility of that bad outcome, they are disappointed and angry and want somebody to blame. Patients can, and sometimes do, with impunity, exaggerate the severity of symptoms.

However carefully a doctor tries to discuss the risks of a procedure, however conscientiously it is documented in the records, a patient can always claim that they do not recall the warning, or did not understand it, or were not given any "insight" into the consequences. The fact is that there is no clinical problem that cannot be made worse by a horrible complication of a procedure; life is a sexually transmitted terminal disease and the only certainty in it is that we are all going to die.

I recall the case of a relatively young ex-soldier who came to me with an infected, multiply revised total knee replacement. We had several lengthy discussions during the time required to assemble all the relevant up to date imaging and microbiology tests. With all the relevant information assembled the management options came down to trying one further major and extremely complex revision, with the possibility of a few more minor operative adjustments subsequently, or going straight to an above knee amputation. We decided to go for a further reconstruction, but I was keen to stress that if that failed badly the only option would   be. . . he interrupted me with a grin and said "I know Doc. It's almost time for me to go out and buy a parrot". Not all patients are like that, but, as far as I know to date, the parrot has not yet been purchased.

The current interpretation of informed consent should probably be abandoned as a justification for litigation. But there is another, relatively simple, form of negligence which cannot be defended; that is incorrect administration of medication; this can take the form either of giving the wrong dose to the right patient or of giving a patient the wrong medication (which would include failing to give prescribed medication).

This is estimated to have cost the NHS £220 million in the last 15 years, £24.3 million last year. More importantly, it is estimated to result in 22,000 deaths each year. Like death, it is a hard outcome from a treatment; either it happened, or it did not. It is a clinical problem, not a legal one. The patient, or their family, deserve compensation, the amount of which will depend on the clinical consequences of the error. Here, as with therapeutic options, the range starts with nothing; that is to say, an acknowledgement, an explanation (trying not to make it sound like an excuse), reassurance that there will be no long-term consequences and an apology, with no financial compensation. I imagine the top of the range, for financial compensation, would be something like killing the high earning young breadwinner for a large young family. There must be some sort of established scale for this, if there is not there should be.

The important and the interesting thing about this form of clinical negligence is the enquiry into how and why it occurred; how did the golf ball get through the tree? Almost always the simple explanation will be staff shortages; exhaustion, loss of concentration, inexperience and inability to find someone to help or check things, unfamiliarity with the drugs cupboard (agency staff), etc. The challenge is how to turn 22,000 events a year into something that is talked about for a hundred years; once again I believe the management strategists are following a flawed plan. They are introducing complex electronic prescription systems and computerized charts for drug administration records, but The NHS IT systems are not sophisticated enough to make these things reproducibly simple to understand and use quickly and reliably. I believe, as I have discussed earlier, the best solution at present lies with improved numbers and quality of staff and the encouragement of teamwork.

The financial cost to The NHS of all this litigation is considerable and rising fast. The reported clinical negligence bill for 2016/17 was £1.08 billion, for 2017/18 £1.63 billion and for 2019 is said to be £2.4 billion. At this time, the total cost of outstanding compensation claims is predicted to be £83 billion, of which £4.3 billion will be legal fees; all this from a total budget for 2019 of £129 billion. The absolute number of litigation cases in recent years has been pretty steady, despite increased clinical activity within the service, but the costs are rising. We live in an increasingly litigious society and anyone who is unhappy with the result of their treatment can allege negligence, encouraged by the lawyers, with, as far as they know at this point, no significant adverse consequences.

But the real cost of litigation is not just financial. It is a very emotionally exhausting and depressing process to go through, both for the claimant and the defendant. I have followed, clinically, patients going through the litigation process on several occasions over many years. Even if their case is fully justified and they stand to get worthwhile compensation they are psychologically unable to put their frustrations behind them until it is closed, which can take many years. Often, long before resolution, they wish they had never embarked on the process, but once started they cannot bring themselves to stop it. What they really need is to accept what has happened and get on with making the best they can of the rest of their lives.

For the defendants, who often feel that they have done nothing wrong, it is also an emotional trauma that is time consuming and physically draining.

There is a school of thought that there should be a bar on patients claiming damages from the NHS, but I do not subscribe to it. Some bad outcomes are clearly more than just bad luck and can have major and irreversible consequences, administering the wrong medication, removing the wrong organ or amputating the wrong limb being simple examples. Any civilized society would wish to see the victim compensated in some way.

Perhaps there is a way to avoid litigation but retain compensation for "injured" patients.

Under the current system all allegations of negligence are referred to a department called NHS Resolution, to which the NHS Trusts pay exceptionally large sums of money as insurance indemnity. Yet less than 2% of the cases referred to NHS Resolution end up in court, the rest being settled by agreement before court, or dropped by the claimant; but by this stage lawyers will have become heavily involved.

The NHS, once again, is paying billions for individuals to make large sums of money; the lawyers, of course; the medical indemnity insurers, of course; those doctors who build up a large practice as expert opinions, without ever being asked to prove whether they are genuine experts or clinical bigots, or both.

The cost of going to court is so high and the courts can be so unpredictable that the safe and cost-effective solution for NHS Resolution is to settle out of court, with no admission of guilt on the part of the defendant, even if the allegation is plainly spurious. Thus, a vexatious litigant is likely to gain some compensation, whether deserving or otherwise.

An alternative and, in my belief, infinitely preferable system is that of "No Fault Compensation", such as exists in New Zealand. A patient who feels they have been the victim of clinical negligence can ask for their case to be reviewed by a Tribunal. This is, in effect, how many litigation cases start already. A disgruntled or unhappy patient asks for their treatment to be reviewed by the relevant clinical management in the form of The Patient Advisory and Liaison Service (PALS), but if they are unhappy with the explanations they receive their only recourse is to go to the Litigation Lawyers, who, of course, welcome them with open arms; the financial floodgates are cranking open.

How much better if they could simply ask for their case to be referred to the Compensation Tribunal, which would be the start and, hopefully virtually always, the finish of the whole negligence compensation process, under the aegis of NHS Resolution.

Remember, this is already what happens in over 80% of negligence allegation cases, but only after a lengthy, grueling and hugely expensive legal process.

The clinicians on the Tribunal would be vetted as people with a genuine experience in the relevant clinical field, all NHS practicing consultants or recently retired Honorary or Emeritus Consultants. The sometimes slightly shady private practice of the Expert Witness would be bypassed, but consultants with a genuine enthusiasm for medico-legal debate could apply to sit on a tribunal as part of their NHS job plan. There should be some lay people chosen from the community of the local tribunal on the most catholic basis and, YES, some lawyers, preferably barristers and judges (possibly again including some recently retired) with some expertise in litigation (not clinical, we hope that will be a thing of the past) settlements. The legal mind is invaluable in this sort of situation, so long as it is not being obliged, professionally, to act in an adversarial fashion.

There could be several tribunals spread around the UK with enough members to always find people with a relevant expertise for each case and ideally each case should be reviewed and resolved by a distant tribunal. The need for live interviews with the claimant and the "defendants" (they are not usually being accused of any failure of duty of care) would, I think, be rare.

The tribunal, if they felt it appropriate, could award a sum in compensation which would be paid by the employing trust, probably through NHS Resolution; but the cost to The NHS would be a fraction of what it is now. If the complainant were unhappy with the outcome, they could appeal to another tribunal elsewhere in the country; but only after that should the possibility of involving the formal judicial systems arise.

If the tribunal found that there had possibly been a genuine and concerning breach of duty of care by the clinicians, they could refer the case to the relevant regulatory body, usually the GMC. My experience is that this would be rare, but at present the courts have no power to do this.

Litigation is invariably emotionally and financially extremely expensive, it should be eliminated.

Compensation can be just and appropriate and should be relatively painless for all concerned.

Medical Malpractice is when a clinician deviates, not only from the accepted standards of their profession, but also in breach of the laws of the land. This is usually for monetary gain, revenge or, most often, for some form of perverted sexual or other psychopathic gratification. It is basically a criminal offence and, although it may come to light through a regulatory body enquiry, it necessitates prosecution through the Criminal Courts.

The NHS and its employees have no role to play other than to give evidence if asked to do so. It should not be a financial burden on the NHS.

Chapter 6
Staffing Agencies

Clinical staffing, particularly for nurses and to a slightly lesser extent doctors, is a chronic (that means long standing although it is sometimes used to imply very bad) and severe problem for the NHS. There are many reasons for this which are best considered in each appropriate chapter, but the fundamental problem has become pay and, perhaps even more significantly, conditions. Most hospitals have a frighteningly high proportion of established nursing posts unfilled, or covered by temporary staff, at any given time. It is impossible to know the exact figures, the data is not collected – let alone released, but I would say somewhere between a quarter and a third of posts; in some locations and departments it is probably very much higher.

There is no slack in the system to cover leave, annual or sick, and whilst no organisation can run efficiently if it is overstaffed there should be close to a full quota of established and experienced staff to deal with the unexpected. The recent coronavirus pandemic has illustrated this perfectly.

This shortage has led to the development of staffing agencies; a huge drain on NHS funds that provides no long-term benefit to health care delivery. The agencies are usually set up by people with some background of NHS employment, but who clearly either do not enjoy frontline clinical work or do not regard the remuneration as sufficient. Qualified nurses and doctors can sign up for an agency which will find them employment either in the NHS clinical front line or in the private sector. This could be anywhere in the country (or indeed, with some agencies, anywhere in the world). The agencies therefore can provide staff at short notice and for this they charge an exorbitant rate. This enables them to pay their staff at a higher rate than an NHS equivalent and still retain a very fat management fee for themselves. The cost to the NHS is enormous and, in some circumstances, up to six times what they would pay for an NHS equivalent qualified doctor, but overall, the cost to the NHS must be many millions a year.

From the point of view purely of income, working for an agency is therefore obviously attractive to clinical staff. It is not difficult to imagine situations where this could be very appealing; a temporary or fairly short-term need for an increase in income, the ability to work for periods to earn money and then have free time, for instance to travel or follow other interests such as a top-class sporting career, but in the longer term working for an agency is essentially a dead-end job. I dare say the employment terms on offer vary from one agency to another but for all of them they can offer no job security, no scope for professional development, and no real professional regulation of knowledge or skills. Some agency staff are highly motivated, knowledgeable and competent and there have recently been many harrowing tales of agency staff contracting and dying from Covid-19, but even the best of them arriving in a new department or ward will take a little time to pick up the structure of the working practices that they need to take up. They are therefore, even if only for a few days, something of a burden on the permanent staff, with no long-term possibility of any benefit to the department or ward.

That is the best that can be said of agency staff, but from my own observation over many years I have no doubt that that represents the minority. Many agency staff are frankly lazy, unreliable people, who want easy money for an easy life. They have no loyalty to the institution to which they have been sent and no interest in maintaining professional standards or partaking in teaching or research.

As they are paid by the hour, they have no interest in efficiency but are happy to work very slowly, which they often do. This is obviously a major source of anger and frustration to the regular NHS employed staff who, effectively, are obliged to carry them and shield them from their own ineptitude in the interests of the patients and the institution for which they work. This is time consuming and reduces the efficiency of the regular staff.

If you are wondering whether or not you enjoy your work, nothing could be more damaging to your morale than starting each shift finding that you have to carry a significant number of incompetents, who are earning twice as much as you are. It just might make one decide to leave a job that had previously been enjoyable.

So how has this ridiculous situation arisen? In the short term, management have put themselves in a position where they have no option but to use agency staff, but why have they created that situation or allowed it to happen? I have often wondered if some managers have an "interest" in a staffing agency and I imagine that some agencies have been set up by ex-NHS managers. Certainly, in the current situation the use of the agencies is the easy solution for managers but that does not make it a good solution. Agency staff are a potential danger to patients but, that of course does not really worry managers as their mantra of "patient safety above all" is, as I have said previously, a lie. The real management motivation is to hit the targets and get the bonus.

The clinical scenario I presented in an earlier chapter, where a consultant anaesthetist pretended, for a joke, to be a vet is, tragically, all too believable. There is a desperate shortage of anaesthetists to cover elective operating lists and the management use agency staff anaesthetists to fill this gap. They have no idea, or any interest in, the competence of the people they are employing. They are happy to accept that they are registered with an agency. I have worked with agency anaesthetists who are palpably incapable of dealing with anything unexpected or difficult in a clinical situation. Happily, knowing that most of my lists were covered by anaesthetists whom I trusted implicitly, I was able to juggle my planned operating to ensure that a "rogue anaesthetist" was not presented with anything that could represent a clinical challenge. I could do this because I was a very senior consultant surgeon with, effectively, nothing to lose. It would have been extremely difficult for a junior colleague to manipulate things in the same way.

I recall one anaesthetist who made so many mistakes and sailed so close to the wind that eventually most of the anaesthetic assistants in the department refused to work with him. Many of the surgeons also refused to undertake lists covered by him. After a great deal of paperwork, it was agreed that he would no longer be employed by The Trust and he returned, without censure, to his agency to wreak his havoc elsewhere.

To my horror, six months later, he was back in that department and I was assured by anaesthetic colleagues that he was then, without any improvement, by no means the worst of the agency anaesthetists now employed by the Trust. The operating lists had been done, the targets were being met and, more by luck than judgement, nobody had been killed or damaged – happy management, stressed and overburdened fulltime clinical teams.

Here is another "possible" clinical scenario. There is a group of clinical staff called Operating Department Practitioners (ODPs). They have trained rather like nurses, but specifically to work in operating departments, either as an assistant to the anaesthetist or somebody who can work as a scrub assistant to the surgeon, or a theatre runner. Within their job descriptions they may be able to take blood, put up drips, draw up drugs as prescribed etc, basically everything that a State Registered Nurse could also do but only within the confines of the operating theatre department.

An agency ODP presents themselves to a theatre department and is one of those people who is an annoying know all but, in fact, knows nothing and has misunderstood most of what they do know. They work for several months within the department on an agency salary engendering an increasing amount of frustration and annoyance. Eventually several anaesthetists refuse to work with them, also a number of the established theatre teams refuse to have them on their shift for the day. At this time a junior theatre manager, desperate for staff, offers this person full time employment, which they accept and so become, without any formal assessment or interview, a full-time member of the NHS staff. This is considered, by every clinician, to be a deplorable mistake, but it ticks a management box in that they have recruited a permanent member of staff.

They continue working for some weeks, incapable and unwilling to learn anything or listen to anybody, until one day they are allocated to work with an anaesthetist covering the case of a young woman with a chronically infected ununited fracture. The anaesthetic and the surgery go well and at the surgeon's request the anaesthetist prescribes an antibiotic called Vancomycin to be administered intravenously in the immediate post-operative period. The OPD goes to the drug cupboard in the anaesthetic room to draw this up and put into an intravenous infusion. Unfortunately, they do not draw up Vancomycin, a commonly used antibiotic which is given by infusion and which, like any antibiotic, can produce allergic reactions, but instead they erroneously draw up a drug called Vecuronium and label the infusion fluid as having been instilled with Vecuronium, which had not been prescribed.

Vecuronium is one of a group of neuromuscular blocking agents. It induces muscle paralysis which can be useful before undertaking an endotracheal intubation of a patient as part of general anaesthesia. Given as a single dose it lasts very effectively but for a short period of time. This group of drugs have a well-documented history of causing catastrophic injuries or death if used inappropriately; in particular, Vecuronium has been used as part of a drug cocktail that prison authorities in the United States use as a means of executing a condemned prisoner. The state security forces of various nations use this drug in interrogation. It is injected into the person being questioned who becomes paralysed and unable to breathe, a bit like drowning. Eventually the prisoner loses consciousness but by then the drug is wearing off and they recover, to be told that this time an antidote has been used to bring them back to life. If they do not co-operate, the next time the antidote will not be given. It must be a very terrifying way of facing death.

Here we have another golf ball being shot through a tree.

Given as an infusion, the drug does not work immediately but accumulates slowly. By the same token, it does not wear off because of the continuous infusion but gradually builds up, so that the patient becomes more and more deeply paralysed, although fully conscious. Because they are progressively unable to breathe their oxygen levels in the blood gradually diminish and they become unresponsive.

Fortunately, this happens on the recovery ward where they are being carefully monitored and observed. One possibility for this dramatic deterioration is that they are having a type of allergic response and therefore all drugs being administered are immediately stopped. The patient is given oxygen, their cardiac function, which has not yet actually deteriorated, is continually checked, they gradually recover and there is no obvious explanation for why they became immobile, unresponsive and unconscious with low blood oxygen. As oxygenation returns to normal the patient becomes responsive and completely well, so the various infusions (being considered part of the important therapy in treating the infection) are restarted.

Half an hour later the same thing happens again. The patient, while maintaining normal cardiac function as monitored, gradually becomes immobile, unresponsive, drowsy and registers a low blood oxygen. Once again, they are appropriately resuscitated but this time the consultant anaesthetist in charge of the recovery unit feels that further investigation is required and checks the labelling on every individual infusion. This reveals that the prescribed antibiotic has probably been replaced by a neuromuscular blocker and a double check on the drug cupboard confirms that to be the case.

The patient makes a full recovery and thanks to the care and skill of the recovery room staff and the investigative intelligence of the anaesthetist in charge no harm has been done, except for the extraordinarily terrifying experience of the patient.

The golf ball has been stopped whilst still in the tree, but the story does not end there.

All the clinicians involved think that, at last, the management must suspend the erring ODP, who has been such an irritant for so many months, pending an enquiry; but no enquiry is called, no investigation is made, no action is taken.

Because the agency ODP had actually been hired by the management without any form of interview or call for references, and because they had been appointed and allowed to proceed to work without the routine of a basic mandatory training being fulfilled, it was clear that any blame for the error must ultimately fall on the management.

So, the whole episode gets swept under the carpet. The ODP continued to work for a few weeks, being very carefully observed by the clinicians around her, before returning to their agency without censure.

Once again, if you think this could not happen, think again and if you think it should not happen you are absolutely right. In this potential situation the management's callous lack of interest in the wellbeing of the patients is exemplified but interestingly, so is their inability to consider the long term, rather than just the short term, consequences of events. What the managers fail to realise is that agency staff are not only a potential danger to patients, but also a danger to the very existence of the institutions for which they are responsible and from which they expect to get their bonuses.

The agency staff are without doubt an absolute danger within the NHS. They provoke inefficiency by failing to turn up just because they don't feel like it, they lead to situations where operating lists are cancelled and the consequences of their general bad practice are multiple and manifest. If a given institution is unhappy with the performance of an agency employee, they can do absolutely nothing about it. They have no means of insisting on them being retrained or monitored in any way. All they can do is get rid of them but, having been moved from one institution they can simply move on and be a danger elsewhere.

This has recently been very tragically illustrated in the investigation of the spread of Covid-19 in care homes. It was found those homes most at danger were those which employed a relatively high proportion of agency staff, who move from one place to another with no fixed commitment and, perhaps, no inclination to feel any sense of responsibility.

So, once again the question arises; here is a problem, can anything be done about it?

In this case the simple answer is yes. What is more, something can be done very easily. The whole concept of agency staff is one of taking advantage of people who have some degree of qualification, or skill, or ability and shunting them into a situation which they may, for short term gain, be seeking, but where the people doing the shunting take the biggest financial gain.

To me this seems like people trafficking. It should simply be declared illegal and stopped absolutely. There is really no need for agencies, but while they exist management will use them.

A mechanism to manage variable demand in staffing levels already exists. Every hospital I have ever worked at has had a "nurse bank"; that is people who are on the permanent staff and have signed up as being willing, if asked, to work extra shifts. All that needs to be done is to deepen the pool of bank nurses. The nurses that now work for agencies are unlikely to leave the profession altogether if the agencies cease. They will take a regular job and if they need more money simply sign on for the nurse bank. People doing extra shifts for the nurse bank should be paid at a noticeably higher rate than the standard one and if money is not thrown away on agencies there would be a great deal more left to pay nurses a respectable wage.

In this way extra staffing needs are met exclusively by people who are already working within the Trust and who have met the Trust's requirements in terms of professional assessment and mandatory training. If somebody moves to another Trust they could remain on the bank of their prior employer and sign up to the bank of their new employer. There could then be a large pool of skilled and experienced workers who are documented and monitored.

In the hospital where I worked there was a wonderful Filipino nurse called, let us say, Nelly. She loved her job, which was really her hobby and her social life. She was happy making herself available through the bank system. As well as working on her own ward she would appear on pretty much every ward in the hospital from time to time and everybody knew her, just as she knew everybody. Every hospital needs more Nellie's.

In order to gear up the bank nursing system it would also be necessary to dramatically improve most Trusts' HR Departments. I have frequently seen the process of staff recruitment blocked by the length of time it took the HR Department to process applicants and clear them for employment. Numerous promising applicants were lost because they were not prepared, or could not afford, to wait for weeks before receiving a contract offer.

This is, of course, all a doubly cunning management plan. Despite the enormous cost of some investigations and treatments the biggest bill facing the managers is the wages bill. Understaffing the HR Department not only saves wages there, but also creates an automatic block meaning that it takes longer to fill replacement posts or create and fill new posts in every department. The wages bill is considered as an ongoing cost that must be monitored and minimised, whereas the fees paid to agencies is considered as a "one of emergency" payment, for which no individual or department is responsible.

So, the wages bill remains lower than it should be and the whole system runs on the goodwill of what staff there are; but goodwill is not a limitless resource. In some parts of the country people simply cannot afford to live on a nurse's salary. By ending the money wasted on agencies, but keeping it in the staff funding pool, nurses could receive a better wage, those that wanted to earn even more could sign up for the bank system and the NHS providers would no longer be exposing themselves to the considerable dangers of agency staff.

Because there are significantly fewer of them, a formal bank system is not necessary for doctors. Short term staffing problems with doctors can usually be covered internally. Longer shortages can be covered by the locum system. A locum (a term only applied to doctors and priests) is filling a post in someone else's place. They are paid no more than the person they are replacing (possibly less) and will have been selected by the institution, not just sent along by an agency. In medicine a locum post is often used by a doctor to find out if they want the post on a permanent basis, or by the institution to check that they want to offer the doctor a permanent post. This system works well.

Chapter 7
Assets to retain or sell

As a public institution the NHS should not be seeking to make an overall profit, but some aspects of its necessary functions could generate income whilst others are inevitably incredibly expensive. Outsourcing some NHS activities is an increasingly common practice, I am really not sure why. No company is going to take on a contract to supply goods or services to anybody unless they think they are going to make a profit from it. Also, people who want to work in a hospital or for a GP practice probably want to identify with and be identified as part of that. They do not want to be on a different contract with a different paymaster. I have already mentioned this in the case of things like portering, cleaning, parking and maintenance. Outsourcing these things may save some administrative costs but surely the NHS is a large enough organisation to absorb the administrative load and any savings are very much at the expense of loss of loyalty within the workforce.

There are two specific functions which have been, or are in the process of being, sold off in circumstances which I think are either a grave mistake or a missed opportunity and I will discuss them in a little more detail.

First, a missed opportunity; catering. NHS food is, quite simply, appalling; it is well known that long term inpatients develop malnutrition syndromes. To some extent it suffers from the need to cater for all tastes, which I have mentioned before, but that should not be an excuse.

Considering inpatients for example, the hospital assumes the responsibility to feed everybody, but why? It would need a change of public expectation, but why shouldn't people who can provide for themselves be encouraged to do so? Feeding everybody inevitably, like all forms of equality, comes down to the lowest common denominator. If over half of the inpatient population was making its own food arrangements (which could be sensibly supervised) then the catering department could focus more attention on specific tastes and requirements of a much smaller number of people. Each ward or unit could have a kitchen set aside for relatives and friends to perhaps heat meals that they had brought in for the patient (I am certainly not suggesting cooking from scratch), but somewhere where soup could be warmed would be useful. In any case, what is wrong with eating cold food. A well-made fresh sandwich is much more nutritious and enjoyable than mash potatoes in cold gravy, soggy elderly Brussel sprouts and an unchewable slice of beef.

Some patients clearly prefer a room of their own, but many prefer to be in, for instance, a single sex four bed bay where they have some company. In that situation perhaps one patient could arrange for his relatives to bring in food for one of the other patients. Clearly it would require some supervision to make sure that nutritious food was being served and hygiene was maintained, but if it worked well, it would improve patients' morale and their nutritional wellbeing.

All this would require a massive change in patient, more particularly their relatives and friends, attitudes to and expectations of the NHS; it certainly could not be switched on "overnight". There would, of course, be enormous demographic variations, with some hospitals having a much higher proportion of patients interested in supplying their own food than others. There would be architectural variations between hospitals for available space to provide facilities for each ward. There would be manpower implications with catering staff having to supervise in-ward services. But catering certainly is not working well at the moment and the logistical challenge of moving some of the catering staff out of a department and onto a ward might not be so complex. It might work very well for the hospital's dietitians trying to ensure an appropriate diet for each patient.

I think it could be achieved if introduced gradually, as part of a general overhaul, of how hospitals provided food for their staff, patients and visitors. Each Trust could select a style and a timescale to suit its particular population and buildings.

For visitors and outpatients many hospitals have a shop run by a League of Friends. These are essentially volunteers, who produce filled rolls and sandwiches and provide some food, making a small profit which goes to amenities for the patients and staff. If the NHS really wants to be a health service, rather than an illness service, why fill the hospital entrances with fast food junk outlets? Why not work in partnership with a good quality restaurant? For instance, if there was a catering school in a local College or University why not have them run a restaurant as part of their student course? I can envisage a situation where a family visiting a relative might choose to book a table for dinner in such a restaurant and regard it as an enjoyable evening out. Staff could be given a small discount if they wanted to have a meal that was more than just a snack on the move.

Second, a grave mistake of outsourcing; the excessive and expensive use of Management Consultancies. I have already discussed what I consider to be management difficulties peculiar to a healthcare delivery service, so it seems extraordinary to me that the people best adapted to deal with these, the most familiar with them, are not recognised to be the full time NHS managers already in post. I have a suspicion that the management consultants are often ex-NHS managers who have set up in private and that the hiring of them is a sort of "jobs for the boys" network; but I could not claim that that is more than a suspicion on my part.

In practice what happens, for instance, is that some staff from the consultancy come into the unfamiliar environment of a hospital, for the first time, to start collecting data that they believe to be relevant to the problem that has been put to them. They then analyse the data in some way or other and come up with some suggestions which are usually totally impractical or counterproductive.

Data that is interpreted inappropriately is worse than useless and I am reminded of a story I used to tell to illustrate the importance of correct interpretation of data.

This is a story which I think highlights the dangers of "misinterpretation of data", a mistake that outside Management Consultancies often make when commissioned, at great expense, to collect and interpret data about NHS performance or efficiency. I used to tell it when speaking at Instructional Meetings sometimes, depending a bit on the nature of the meeting and the mood of the delegates and faculty. To satisfy the demands of Political Correctness I have rendered it Nationality, Race, Colour, Creed, Gender and Sexuality neutral. I hope it still seems amusing.

"There were three great friends who met regularly on a Friday evening for a drink and a chat. One evening one of them was particularly late arriving and, on eventually appearing, they looked quite worried and distressed. Asked what was wrong by the first two their friend replied, "I'm really worried about my relationship with my partner; I think they're having an affair with a plumber". The other two expressed their surprise and concern and asked what could have led to this conclusion. The reply came, "Well, it could explain why I keep finding plumber's tools and bits if copper pipe and ballcocks and things under the bed". The three agreed that it did not look good and all expressed a hope that things would work out all right.

About a month later another of the three arrived late and looking distressed. On enquiry the reply came, "I think my partner is having an affair with a carpenter. It's the only thing I can think of to explain why I keep finding wood shavings and saws and planes and things under the bed". Again, there was a general expression of surprise and concern and a hope that all would be resolved.

Another month or so passed and then the third one arrived late and looking very angry. When asked what was wrong the reply came, "I'm leaving my partner. They're having an affair with a horse". The first two friends expressed astonishment and some disbelief, to which the incandescent reply came, "Well how else would you explain why I keep finding a jockey under the bed".

If you think that is too stupid to be true you are, of course, correct; but here is an example of a judgement that I think is comparably stupid and is true.

This involves the efficient use of operating theatre time. An operating facility is extremely expensive to construct, maintain, and staff. Like any plant it should be used as efficiently as possible, but an estimate of how long any operation will take can only be just that, an estimate. There are too many variables:

- the time it takes the ward or theatre admissions unit to prepare a patient for theatre, some control - subject to staffing levels, unexpected other nursing commitments
- several theatres all sending for patients at the same time etc.
- availability of porters, some control
- the patient who wishes to visit the lavatory at the last moment, no control at all
- anaesthetic time, some control in that you can predict the cases that are definitely going to be difficult, but no control over the ones that should be straightforward but become difficult, for all sorts of reasons, including training of junior staff
- operating time, surgeons are notoriously and arrogantly optimistic about how quick they will be – myself included. One should never say (particularly

for complex or unusual procedures) "this will be an easy operation"; only, if appropriate, "that was an easy operation".

That is just for one operation. Imagine an eight-hour list with four major operations planned.

Theatre timings will inevitably over-run their allocation on occasions and, equally will sometimes under-run.

A Management Consultant team was brought in to look at the time lists finished and assess the over-run and under-run times in a unit of eight individual theatres. Over what was considered to be a representative period of time the total underrun for the unit was greater than the overrun by an average of sixteen hours per week. Their stunning conclusion was that the clinical staff in each theatre were wasting a total of two hours of valuable theatre time per week.

As a group the clinicians were accused of "wasting" eight major operations a week in the struggle to meet waiting list targets.

Two hours over five days averages twenty-four minutes a day. Some finishes will have been earlier than that and some days there may have been an over-run, but planning cannot be precise and in any case twenty minutes is not sufficient time to perform even the most minor operative procedure.

They simply did not collect and analyse the appropriate data for assessing theatre efficiency.

For instance, were there particular surgical teams who consistently under-ran, if so why? Much more relevant and useful data to review, but not what the Consultancy was asked to do, or had the insight to think of itself.

This is the sort of meaningless information that the NHS is paying vast sums of money to Management Consultancies to obtain.

Another example of unproductive outsourcing is probably the most pernicious of all. This is primarily a political initiative and therefore it is embraced by the mangers, but sadly it is also supported quite enthusiastically by some of the consultant clinical staff.

It is the practice of effectively buying time in private hospitals to perform operations or investigative procedures.

What happens is this; The NHS contracts and pays a private provider to undertake a number of procedures such as MRI scans or joint replacements. They then pay the local NHS clinicians undertaking the work in the private facility a sum of money to perform it. Their work must be done outside their NHS contracted hours. It is attractive to the politicians and managers because they can boast that they have reduced the numbers on a waiting list by the amount of the contract. It is attractive to some clinicians because it is, in effect, a form of private practice and supplements their NHS salary.

But it is an ill-considered scheme with some serious drawbacks and risks, for training and research, for clinical continuity, one of the essential elements of patient safety and for financial consequences in the longer term.

The private facilities will only undertake operations that are straightforward, on patients with no co-morbidities. Those are clinically low risk patients, who are likely to only require a short in-patient stay and will be easy to discharge.

One of the obligations of all doctors, enshrined in the Hippocratic Oath (although nobody has physically sworn the Hippocratic Oath for many years), is to pass on wisdom and experience – teaching. The sort of cases that are now being done by consultants in private hospitals are exactly the sort of cases that it would be appropriate for teaching trainee surgeons, under supervision, to improve their surgical skills.

In some Trusts virtually all the straightforward elective operations are being done by consultants in private hospitals as NHS patients. The consultants are paid extra for a bit of extra work, but the training opportunity is lost. All that is done at the NHS hospitals are the complex cases, such as revisions, which it would not be appropriate, or even safe, to allow the trainees to undertake from start to finish for practical experience. They may be allowed to observe and take some part, but they cannot do the major part or learn to make intra-operative decisions themselves. Often the trainees are told that they are not insured to undertake any clinical activity in the private

hospital, so they cannot even observe; or they may have some other NHS clinical commitment which prevents them.

The training of doctors includes involving them in research projects and outcome studies. The NHS makes a major contribution to global clinical knowledge and all the cases that have been sequestered into the private sector are much more difficult, if not impossible, to include in these types of study.

We are producing a generation of trainees who will only have acquired limited surgical skills by the time they should be considering becoming a consultant and taking on their own independent practice.

The NHS is selling off those cases from which a private facility believes it can make a profit and is being left only doing the complex cases, either because of technical difficulties or because of multiple co-morbidities. These are the patients that require longer inpatient stays postoperatively and become increasingly more and more expensive.

It might sound as though this is a win/win situation for the patients. They get their treatment in a private hospital and their surgery will be undertaken by a consultant. Likewise, interventional radiology will be performed by a consultant, not a supervised (possibly from a distance) trainee. The NHS picks up the bill. For most treatment episodes this is what happens, but that does not necessarily mean that it is a better or safer option; nothing focuses the mind like teaching another person and resident junior medical cover in private hospitals often leaves a lot to be desired.

There is also a group that fall through this net into a limbo of frustration and delay. I am not quite sure why, but in this so-called "choose and book system" patients can be seen significantly sooner with an appointment in a private hospital than they can in the mainstream NHS hospital. Most GPs will screen their patients to make sure that they significant co-morbidities such as obesity or ...opulmonary disease, but the lure of a relatively early appointment is strong. There are a small number of GPs who feel that this fast-track is the best way to serve their patients and may not have any insight into the potential pitfalls.

The patient is then seen, say for an arthritic knee, by a consultant surgeon who might recommend a knee replacement to be done in the private hospital. There is still some waiting time for the operation and the patient is not seen again until they receive an appointment for a pre-operative assessment with an anaesthetist.

At this point they may be rejected as not "safe" to be operated on in the private hospital.

This could be a clinical judgement; possibly a difference of opinion between surgeon and anaesthetist about, for instance, obesity; perhaps some medical condition that the surgeon had not picked up, like an abnormal heart rhythm; or something may have changed between the two consultations, a new co-morbidity.

It could also be a financial judgement; if the patient is going to be difficult to discharge, they could cost the hospital more than the tariff they will be paid for the procedure.

"Safe" is not just about patient welfare, it is also about profitability.

Whatever the reason the patient, thinking they have been on an accelerated and possibly preferable pathway, suddenly finds themselves back at the start of the process for treatment.

The surgeon might refer the patient to a colleague, or even himself, in the NHS, but then the NHS might reject the referral on the grounds that it has not been made by a GP. Technically the patient has been referred for consideration of operative treatment and turned down. Sometimes the patient is left erroneously thinking that surgery is not an option for them. Even if they manage to get into the NHS system the "target" rules mean that their waiting time does not start until the date of the referral letter to the NHS hospital that is planning the surgery. So, although the system works for many people there are some who are left frustrated and angry.

Another aspect of the double standards of the system is the question of who picks up complications. Usually, the contract with the private provider has some clause to say that complications up to thirty days or three calendar months will be picked up by the private provider but anything that happens after that inevitably becomes a problem for the NHS to address. Even before that time there are some surgical complications which private hospitals, in most cases, are simply not equipped to deal with and these would have to be transferred to the NHS hospital as well.

So, the supposedly, easy operation has gone wrong, for whatever reason, but the profit from doing it, possibly badly, has gone to the private sector. The enormous cost of trying to put it right is left to the NHS.

I will consider the general standards of safety in private hospitals in Chapter 10.

In these various ways I believe that The NHS is selling off "assets" which it would be in its interests to retain. It is also retaining assets which it could usefully sell or turn to more profitable effect.

The smooth field (Smithfield) outside the city walls of London was a good place for a hospital in 1172 AD, but things have changed. Access is difficult, there is no parking or resident population and the value of the land is astronomical. It is good to maintain important historical sites in their original style, but not necessarily for their original purpose. I would not like to see the Tower of London site sold for a property developer to pull it down and put up a tower-block hotel, but I would not want it still used for its original purpose, which was to incarcerate political prisoners and carry out public executions.

Similarly, I cannot really see the sense of having an internationally famous and important children's hospital remaining in the centre of London, one of the busiest cities in the world. It may have been founded there and it is convenient for Harley Street, but the service should be located on a site that is easily accessible by road, rail and air with on-site subsidised accommodation for families. The forces of medical conservatism and personal interest are powerful ones when it comes to resisting change, but Bevan managed to overcome them.

That is just two examples in London, where land values are highest, but there must be hundreds of other examples all around the UK.

I am not suggesting that these sites should all be sold, but I do think that they could be more profitably used as revenue generators to augment NHS funding. I have heard that the Church of England Commissioners sold off large numbers of beautiful vicarages and Georgian rectories when they were worth several hundred thousand pounds each, only to find that, within a very short space of time, they had become worth several million pounds and that, if it is true, was a mistake.

I would not want the NHS to fall into that error.

Chapter 8
Nurse Recruitment and Retention

There has, apparently, been a three-fold increase in people interested in a career in nursing since the Coronavirus pandemic. That surprises me but it must be a good thing if it is sustained. I suspect it will tail off quite quickly, but whether it does or not there needs to be some major changes in the structuring of nurse training, career progression, working environment and remuneration. Much of that restructuring would, in fact, just be a return to the former established ways which worked very well.

Probably more than any other profession or trade, nursing is a vocation and very much a hands-on activity. During the first half of the last century it was almost exclusively a profession for young women, drawing upon widely diverse social and cultural backgrounds. In the second half and the beginning of this century it began to appeal increasingly to young men, which diversity should only have strengthened the profession and increased its popularity. Sadly, that has not really been the case, I think because of several important changes in the training program.

To be a competent nurse requires a fair amount of factual knowledge and, as with every aspect of human endeavour that can only really be acquired by studying, at least in the first instance. To succeed in some professions that is by far the most important attribute, but to be an outstanding nurse, as so many of our NHS nurses are, requires much more than just knowledge. It requires humility, humanity and compassion. It also requires that intangible concept of wisdom. To be wise on any subject requires a combination of knowledge, experience and judgement and of these, knowledge alone is the only one that can be gained from studying books. To be a good nurse, indeed, perhaps to be any kind of nurse at all, requires all these skills and attributes to a greater or lesser extent, but it does NOT necessitate an academic degree.

The New Labour government of 1997 decided, on who knows what basis, that all children had not only "the right", but also "the desire" to go to university. That was confusing "equality of opportunity" with "equality of outcome", a common error made by misguidedly idealistic people attempting social engineering. The first is an ideal that our society should strive to achieve but imposing the second can only be achieved by accepting the lowest common denominator, reductio ad absurdum, very totalitarian. The result was that every Technical College became a University, prestigious for the staff, and every apprenticeship became a degree course, awfully expensive and a waste of time for the apprentices.

I imagine that a group of Nationally influential senior nurses felt that their own prestige would be enhanced if nursing became perceived as an academic pursuit, but this profound misconception has been disastrously damaging to the profession.

Today's students entering a school of nursing spend the vast majority of their three-year course in lecture theatres or writing dissertations, largely, I suspect on subjects which are, at best, very tangential to the provision of good nursing care. An example might be, how to interact with patients without offending them. This is a problem littered with pitfalls, the avoidance of which is not guaranteed by any amount of theoretical preparation. I recall two incidents involving elderly gentlemen which could never have been foreseen, but where, of course, no harm was done because the "interactions" were well intended and sympathetic.

One involved a Peer of the Realm whose personal details stated that his given name was Tony. A student nurse said to him, on the way to the operating theatre, while he was probably a little apprehensive, "What would you like us to call you, Tony". He snapped back "Your Lordship". The other was someone who employed a very loyal valet from a particular military background. He was being shown how to get out of bed following his operation and used the pole projecting from the head of the bed for assistance. A nurse said to him "You will have to learn to do it without the pole. You won't have a pole at home". He replied, in annoyed astonishment, "I don't need a Pole. I've got a Gurkha".

Perhaps learning how to address patients is best done by addressing patients, who will exhibit an infinite variety of personalities in infinitely variable circumstances.

University-type courses are an expensive process for the student involved. I have no doubt that people who would love to pursue a career in nursing are deterred from starting it by the thought of those three years and the eventual debt that it might incur.

Perhaps the solution, as is so often the case, would be to return to the way things were before any of this fantasy social revolution was thrust upon us. Nurse training was essentially a prestigious apprenticeship. Most towns or cities with a sizable General Hospital and all the Teaching Hospitals would have their own School of Nursing, which should now be linked to a nearby University. In tandem, and according to National Standards, they would supervise the school as a discrete faculty on the hospital site. This faculty would be run on a daily basis by nurse teachers, nurses who had gone into education as their chosen sub-specialisation.

Formal lectures would be given on site by the clinical staff of the hospital; there might, at most, be a small honorarium for this, but ideally a commitment to teach should be included as a part of all clinicians contracts. Spending 40 minutes or an hour talking to students is something that most clinicians find very enjoyable and rewarding.

But the major part, at least two thirds, of the curriculum should be time that the students spend in the wards and clinical departments of the hospital. They would be supervised by the established Staff Nurses and Sisters and would thus be experiencing, and gradually gaining expertise in, the practical techniques and skills of clinical nursing. As they progressed through the course the supervision would become more and more of a light touch and they would acquire the ability and the confidence to manage clinical situations independently.

In addition, as they came towards the end of their course, they would realise that they knew, and were known by, many of the hospital staff. They might dislike that very much, but it is far more likely that they would feel part of a "family", a team. They would be comfortable dealing with doctors, who can be "difficult" (remember the manure analogy), and would, hopefully, identify very positively with the institute that had trained them. On qualifying as a State Registered Nurse, they would be far more likely to seek a substantive post in the hospital, or at least within the NHS, rather than drift off into some better remunerated activity.

All Schools of Nursing should provide student nurses with accommodation in an on-site Nurses Home. Accommodation in the Home, at a cost, should ideally be available to junior or transient qualified clinical staff, but for the student nurses it should be at least heavily subsidised, preferably, free. Long gone are the days when a student nurses' home could be equated to a girls' school dormitory. Nursing now attracts a large and diverse group of individuals from a wide range of socially, culturally and ethnically different backgrounds. Without that varied contribution from, for example, Asian, Afro-Caribbean and Filipino communities the NHS would probably have ceased to exist many years ago. They all share the same hopes and aspirations and are all, I believe, treated the same; the staffing of the NHS is really a shining example of equal opportunity in our society. Such a community can only be a good thing.

Not only should the student nurses be accommodated and welcomed within the hospital, but they should also be salaried, because of the work they would be doing on the wards and in the various clinical departments. They would be far more reliable, useful and enthusiastic than most of the agency staff currently employed. The salary need not be large, but it should be sufficient to enable all but the most profligate of students to qualify without having incurred a significant debt. It would still save a lot on the wages bill compared to the use of agencies.

Suddenly, in my opinion, being a student nurse is beginning to look rather attractive. Perhaps there would be a competitive element to gaining a place in a School of Nursing, just as there is to the great Universities and Medical Schools.

Prior to the pseudo-intellectualising of nursing at the turn of the century there was a second, very productive, pathway into the profession; The State Enrolled Nurse. As far as I recall this was a simplified apprenticeship type training without so much of the more formal educational aspects. They acquired all the practical skills of working in a ward or department, fulfilling an especially useful role in training, for which they were paid just like those training to become a registered nurse.

They wore a slightly different uniform, but I do not believe that most patients recognised the distinction, they were all just addressed as nurse. They might be people whose children had grown up and who had looked for a career a little later in life, but they could well have already developed the sympathy and compassion which are such a vital aspect of nursing. They could not administer or distribute medications, but they had the potential to become highly skilled in technical procedures, according to each individual trust, such as taking blood samples and putting up intravenous lines. There was the possibility of doing a conversion course to become a Registered Nurse if they wished, but in any case, they also had the potential to advance their career in basically the same way as a State Registered Nurse, although they would be starting from a slightly less qualified perspective.

I believe it would be hugely beneficial to reinstate that pathway, probably with the same title of State Enrolled Nurse. I can see no reason why it was ever stopped; perhaps just an unnecessary attempt to enhance the prestige of the title "nurse".

Strong recruitment and good staff retention are equally important for developing an experienced and fulfilled clinical workforce. My thoughts on retention of nursing staff apply just as much to other clinical staff, physiotherapists, occupational therapists, radiographers, etc. All these vital clinicians can become disillusioned with the environment and remuneration of NHS employment.

Salaries are, undoubtedly, an important factor, although it is more of a problem in specific regions where the cost of living is high. They are ridiculously low for the level of skill, responsibility and dedication that the work involves. Successive governments have cynically taken advantage of the clinicians' natural reluctance to withhold their labour and that must change. It would not be difficult to pay more if less money was wasted on agencies, but it is also important to provide a good career path, with incentives of increased remuneration with increasing seniority, experience and responsibility.

At present the only way to move up the career ladder and the salary scale is, basically, to abandon direct clinical care and move into management. This is an option which is unattractive or even unacceptable to many. Perhaps the career pathways could be restructured into several different routes, so that being drawn further and further into management is no longer the only way to increase status and salary.

In hospitals for instance a senior staff nurse working on a ward might aspire to be the ward "sister", which is an important and responsible role. At present it involves spending more and more time off the ward in meetings, but perhaps the role could be changed so that more time was spent on the wards supervising and teaching. Wards could hold their individual budgets and the individual ward leaders ("sisters") could manage those, but they would not be expected to absent themselves from the clinical practice. Becoming more senior and experienced in organising wards could lead to a clinical advisory role for other wards with remuneration appropriate to the experience and valuable contribution to the hospital's clinical practice.

The same pattern could be applied to nurses working in operating theatres. The more senior and experienced they become the more useful they are in the theatre environment, but the only way to improve their grade on the salary scale is, effectively, to remove themselves from that environment where they are at their most useful. They should be rewarded for their work in the clinical front line, not forced to move "out of department" as the only way to enhance their salary.

I have no personal experience of it, but I imagine the same pattern applies to nurses working in the community.

Other nurses and therapists become fascinated by clinical research or even sometimes basic science research. It is widely acknowledged that they are far more meticulous collectors of data than doctors. People on that career pathway make an invaluable contribution to clinical activities as well as to the research. They might want to take a degree or even a postgraduate qualification such as a master's degree or a doctorate and they should be encouraged to do that if they wish to. The cost should be covered by the hospital or community employers.

Progress in clinical medicine is based on evidence and evidence is based on the collection of data, whether it be data about the efficacy of a medication or data about the performance and longevity of a prosthetic implant. The more time they spend collecting data the better they will become and the greater the contribution they will be able to make to its interpretation. Misinterpretation of data can lead to bizarre conclusions, but in clinical medicine a bizarre conclusion is not funny, it can be extremely damaging or even fatal. There is a potentially huge role for nurses and therapists in this field and the more they contribute the more they should be paid.

Other nurses and therapists wish to develop specialist interests without necessarily partaking in the research aspects. Again, there is a large and probably increasing need for this kind of specialisation. For many years I ran my practice with specialist physiotherapists who saw patients in clinic, both to list them for surgery and to review them postoperatively. These people were of far more use to me, and more importantly to my patients, than any junior doctor could ever be because they became a longstanding part of the team rather than being moved on every six months. They were more accessible to patients than the doctor can be, particularly a busy GP or hospital consultant, but they have direct access to the doctor in charge of the patient's overall clinical care. This role ranges from mental health, through social and community care and musculoskeletal disease to the diagnosis and management of cancers. Therapists and nurses who wish to go into that kind of work should be remunerated as they become more senior and experienced and therefore more useful. More useful than junior doctors, but the junior doctors are also there as part of their training programme.

There will always be a role for clinicians who want to go into clinical management and so there should be. Just as there are doctors who do not particularly want to spend time with patients, so there are nurses who prefer to develop skills in strategic planning and management, they are very necessary. They too should be able to take additional qualifications to help with their professional development and something like a master's degree should be paid for by the institution.

I put these suggestions forward just as an idea, each professional clinical group should know best what would work for them. But some way must be found to provide nurses and therapists with a fulfilling and financially rewarding career structure that does not obligate them to preparing reports and attending meetings, unless that is specifically what they choose to do.

Retention of staff is not, of course, just about progressive financial remuneration. It is equally, if not more importantly, about creating a working environment that is attractive and emotionally rewarding. Mark Twain apparently said, with great insight, "find a job you enjoy doing and you will never have to work a day in your life". There are many things that make a job enjoyable, colleagues, teams, environment, respect, accessibility, to name a few. They are all interacting. Teamwork for instance will lead to a lessening of intimidation (bullying), support (the opposite of isolation), fulfilment (the opposite of frustration). Similarly, there are many aspects of environment, but I believe that an important one is opportunities for social interactions at work. Hospitals used to be a community, with enormous scope for socialising in a friendly and enjoyable atmosphere. When I first went to the hospital where I worked for nearly forty years there were, within the grounds, three tennis courts, a hall with badminton courts which could be hired for dances and private functions, a heated swimming pool with a lifeguard and a bar that would serve food and drinks. All of that was perhaps particularly privileged, but many hospitals would have some form of Sports and Social Club. All these facilities have now gone; partly because of changes in the broader society, but mainly because they were space occupying and expensive to maintain. Nevertheless, I think it would be a good thing to restore them in some form. This could go hand in hand with the reintroduction of nurses' homes and onsite accommodation. Space for socialising is always the first thing on the managers' list to be sacrificed, but I think it should not be that way. Space for socialising should be regarded as a valuable and important facility.

Finally, perhaps the most important factor that would help with staff retention also relates to space, on-site childcare facilities. A large proportion of hospital staff have young families, with both parents working full time. In many ways a hospital is in a perfect position to provide nursery and junior care, which should of course be free, or at the very least heavily subsidised, for staff. The salaries of many of the lower paid clinical workers would not even cover the cost of childcare. Unfortunately, it represents a long-term investment when the overwhelming priority is simply to hold back the financial firewall; managers do not really have the option to think in the longer term.

There are ways in which individual Hospital Trusts and Community Trusts could generate some income for their own use. Surely one of the best ways to spend it would be in enriching the working environment and improving staff retention and loyalty. I have talked about reducing expenditure by abolishing agencies and outsourcing of work. I will talk about the generation of income in Chapter 11.

Chapter 9
Doctor Recruitment and Retention

Recruitment of students to Medical Schools is not really a problem in terms of numbers. It is probably not as popular a subject as it was twenty years ago, for various reasons, but it remains in very high demand.

The difficulty, in terms of recruitment for medical school, is to try and determine what aspects of an applicant's abilities might predict that they would go on to make a good, successful and contented doctor. It is, of course, difficult to define what constitutes a good, successful and contented doctor in the first place. It could be defined as a person who continues to practice in that career, in the environment provided by the nation that provided their training, until an appropriate age for retirement; but that is a retrospective observation not a predictive marker. So, the question arises, are the Medical Schools selecting the appropriate candidates. Given that it is an impossible judgement to make, the answer is very likely to be not in all cases, may be not in the majority of cases.

One thing is certainly true, that is that to get through Medical School successfully you must be able to assimilate a very large amount of factual knowledge, much more so than in Nursing School. You then must be able to produce it on demand in an organised and rational form. In other words, a medical student must be good at passing exams, both written and oral. The exams themselves are not a particularly reliable way of assessing an individual's intelligence. Like universal enfranchisement in a democracy, it is accepted because there does not seem to be any better option, but there is no evidence that it produces a particularly desirable outcome. Also, there is no reliable way of assessing the potential for acquisition of attributes like wisdom and fulfilment.

These can only be assessed retrospectively, so exam results have become the overwhelming criteria for success in applying to a Medical School and other admirable characteristics, which are difficult to evaluate, have become increasingly ignored. Worse than that, in some instances, evidence of outstanding ability outside the field of passing exams may have become a reason for rejecting a candidate, on the basis that such interests as sport, music, drama, for instance, may be a distraction from the primary need, which is to acquire knowledge and prove it by passing exams.

It was not always that way. When I applied to Medical School, I was interviewed by the two institutions which I had placed first and second on my application choices. I was interviewed first by my second choice, which entailed being seated in front of a desk behind which were ranged about a dozen interviewers, with no form of introduction other than me confirming my identity. They asked me three questions. The first was, "is your father a doctor?" My answer was no and that was the end of that question. The second was, "if you did come here would you want to continue playing rugby?" My answer was yes and that was the end of that question. The third question was, "why are we your second choice not your first choice?" My answer was (I had been warned of the possibility of this question by a very thoughtful master at my school) to discuss a few differences in their academic requirements and pastoral care. I was thanked and dismissed. They offered me a place.

At the time I thought it was rather a peremptory interview when there was so much at stake for me and my future aspirations. In retrospect I think it was rather an astute and efficient interview. I had already passed the required examinations to a standard which showed a clear ability to acquire knowledge and prove it. They wanted to look for something beyond that and chose topics that they considered relevant; I now think that they made reasonable choices, but I have no regrets that I subsequently accepted a place and attended my first choice.

Let us consider some of the other attributes which might be predictive of who will become a "good" doctor.

Being the child of a medical family is a good measure of whether or not you have some insight into what it entails, I believe there are studies that have shown it to be a useful indicator of leading to a "successful and contented" career.

I consider myself to have been well educated and I certainly feel fortunate to have been the recipient of that opportunity. In my youth I was definitely, when motivated, good at passing exams – what a creep. But I am convinced that the vast majority of the specific and detailed factual knowledge that I needed to pass those exams made virtually no direct contribution to whatever abilities I may have developed and utilised over forty years of practicing clinical medicine and surgery. Perhaps the sheer discipline of learning is, in itself, a useful exercise. But history has shown us that Education and the accumulation of great wealth are not intimately intertwined, and neither is particularly associated with the acquisition of wisdom.

The Victorian explorer, adventurer and "colonialist" Cecil Rhodes created for himself vast wealth and power. The means by which he did so are now widely despised and are certainly not acceptable to the contemporary "free" world. But much of the world is not free by our terms and much of the behaviour of our adventuring forebears, up to the nineteenth century, is still in practice today in other societies. I feel it is a mistake to judge anyone, retrospectively, outside the morals and beliefs of the historical era and society in which they lived, strived and died. All we can do, as always, is to learn from the past and try not to be supportive of those nations which refuse to progress.

To me the interesting thing about Rhodes is not how he acquired his money, but what he did with it preparatory to his death.

Despite his strong association with The University of Oxford he could not consider himself a well-educated man; he only spent one term "in statu pupillari", but it must have influenced him profoundly and enduringly. However he behaved in Southern Africa he had a strong belief that Britain should be a leader in the "enlightenment" of the world and he chose to enable that through the power of education and the English language. Nobody who has any knowledge of The Rhodes Foundation and the Postgraduate Scholarships it awards in Oxford can doubt their prestige and value to those who win them. Initially they were available, competitively, not only to those whose nations were part of The Empire at the time, but to those whose administrative language was English. Thus, the single nation that has probably provided more Rhodes Scholars that any other is the USA, which had made its dislike of the British Empire abundantly clear well over a century earlier. The interesting exception was Germany, where there were historical reasons for admiring their university systems at that time. They are now available to all nations.

Rhodes himself laid down three specific selection criteria, each of which must be met by any candidate; good academic ability, they had to have played representative sport of some kind and they had to have done some voluntary work to the benefit of their community. I understand that these criteria are still a requirement and I hope that they remain so for centuries to come. Rhodes also stated something to the effect that "no candidate shall be accepted or rejected purely on the grounds of race or colour". He may have been a bad man by our contemporary standards but, in my opinion, he seems to have had some very good ideas.

Being good at sport is a useful and reliable indicator of personal ambition, an ability to organise your time and commitments, an ability to contribute within a team structure, and an ability to communicate and socialise. Contributing to the wellbeing of a community shows compassion and consideration as well as selflessness. All these attributes are useful, if not essential, to a successful career in clinical medicine; certainly, more so than following a career, for instance, in banking or the law.

They have now become subjugated, in the selection process, to simple exam performance; I think that is a pity. It may in part explain why some medical students, after a long and arduous period of training to be a doctor, never actually take up the profession, or leave it at the first opportunity. Comparatively recently some Universities have set up an accelerated programme of training to qualify as a doctor, solely for graduates in other subjects. It is just a personal observation, but I have always found these graduate entrants to be outstanding in terms of character, sympathy, ability, motivation, insight, and many other admirable characteristics.

Perhaps aspiring politicians should not be considered as parliamentary candidates unless they have undertaken some meaningful and successful career outside politics first, but that would have ruled out Nye Bevan.

Whether or not there are flaws in the selection processes of candidates for places in Medical Schools, the fact is that the majority of graduating medical students do go on to post-graduate training in clinical medicine, requiring some postgraduate qualifications. There is probably no subject on a university syllabus that more closely predicts the eventual career path of the people reading it and a university education, in any case, is not really about predicting a particular career; for most people it is about learning life skills, including those which will enrich them (in the most catholic sense of the word) for any future career.

It is, however, my strong impression that most doctors, still practicing in the UK, at around twenty years after their post graduate qualification have become increasingly disillusioned with their career pathways and professional environment. That impression is supported by the rate at which they are seeking early retirement; faster than NHS Pension Services can keep up with the applications. It is interesting to speculate why that might be, but this did not happen to me. I enjoyed my job, on the whole, although with some increasing frustrations, right up to the point of my slightly reluctant retirement, but I think that I was extraordinarily fortunate with the environment in which I worked (that is, the particular hospital, the speciality, and most of my colleagues) and with the support of my family. As I planned for retirement, with the handover of my clinical responsibilities and patients requiring ongoing follow-up, every colleague I spoke to, without exception, expressed envy that I was leaving, usually with the added observation that I was escaping just before things became really intolerable. That was months before anybody had ever heard of Covid19.

With nurses and therapists, I genuinely believe that the salary is a major factor in their discontent. Nurses leave to follow other professions and therapists tend to go into private practice. In real terms, doctors' salaries have fallen significantly in the last twenty years (for the same cynical political reasons that nurses' salaries have fallen), but most doctors probably still feel that they are reasonably well paid, although there is probably not a single country in the western world where doctors are not much better remunerated.

I think that the frustrations for doctors are mainly those associated with the working environment. There must be some who would be content to continue to be treated as they are if they were paid more, but I think most would prefer to leave the salary as it is and have better control of their working lives. I have already written about the rather bullying management style, but one effect is that there is constant pressure on the clinicians to see more patients and "perform" better in management metrics. The numbers of patients are simply too great for the numbers of doctors and, to give a simple example, clinics are consistently overbooked on management instructions, despite consultants' requests not to do this. It is extremely stressful trying to complete a clinic when you are halfway through the listed patients and already running two hours late. This stress can be dissipated a little by a good clinical team, but remember that the management do not like teams.

I should now confess, rather sadly, that a lot of clinical "lists" (lists to see a GP, hospital clinic lists, lists for investigations, lists for out-patient treatments, operating theatre lists) do run late, or even end with a few cancellations, but forced overbooking by managers is probably not the most significant cause. Some consultants consistently arrive late for the start of their clinical commitment. I do not know what proportion of staff are guilty of this, I am not aware of any formal collection of the data but speak to any nurse or clerk who runs any list and they will be able to name the culprits with unerring reliability. There are not many of these cheats, for that is what they are, but their influence is far greater and more insidious than their mere numbers. I understand that falsifying a time sheet or expenses claim is a criminal offence; I have never understood why signing a job contract committing to a certain number of clinical hours work and consistently failing to perform them is not considered in the same way.

In any situation where a "workforce" can be assessed for their "productivity" there is a consistent mathematical model (which works!) that can be applied by management wishing to increase productivity. Most workers, say 95%, will be close to the average production. A small number will produce more and a small number very much less. The under-productive ones (the lazy and the cheats) will be difficult to improve and even more difficult to get rid of, so forget them. The very productive ones are probably working as hard as is possible, so forget them, but a small improvement from the 95% will have a big effect on output, so lean on them.

It works in a factory, so it is what is attempted to be applied to clinicians in the NHS. But what this model fails to appreciate is the overwhelmingly dispiriting effect that it has on the majority of NHS clinicians (the 95%) who genuinely want to work efficiently and with a strong commitment to the wellbeing of their patients.

I have already written about consultant job plans and the changing ways in which they are constructed by management. Now, with each newly appointed consultant a less attractive contract is created than was held by his predecessor; more clinical sessions, but specifically not as part of a regular clinical team; less, or no, time allowed for other important aspects of the role – teaching, research, clinical administration, etc.; restrictive annual leave and no study leave allowance. Now, committed consultants also feel that they are carrying the lazy, the incompetent and the cheats; it was ever thus and always will be, but in the old days at least one had an agreeable work pattern oneself.

Worse than just carrying the cheats, the efficient and enthusiastic often find that they are actively blocked, by them, in attempting to provide a good clinical service. This problem is probably best exemplified by considering the organisation of operating theatre lists, the central core of any surgeon or anaesthetist's clinical activity.

To operate on a succession of patients over a day, in a safe and efficient way, requires the coordinated input of quite a large number of individuals or groups of people; lead surgeon and theatre nursing team, lead anaesthetist and anaesthetic assistants, obviously; but also hospital porters, theatre orderlies, theatre receptionists, recovery nurses, ward nurses to prepare the patients for theatre and receive them back from recovery, planning to allow staff breaks without a delay between cases, etc. It sounds complicated but is quite simple and reliable if everyone is keen to achieve the same end, pulling in the same direction.

But it only takes one individual to be out of step for the whole day to fall apart. In my experience the most common breakdowns are at the start of the list and are caused by either the surgeon or the anaesthetist.

Some surgeons, I do not think anyone counted them, but enough to make it obvious in the weekly activities of any complex of four or more theatres, routinely arrive late for their lists. There may be many reasons for this, some operate on private patients the day before and start the day doing a post-operative ward round in the private hospital (breach of contract?) some take their children to school (poor "family planning"), but none of them are acceptable. With anaesthetists the likely cause is reversed (family more frequent than avarice) but one can also add poor motivation, otherwise known as laziness. Most operating lists are scheduled to start (referred to as "knife to skin") at 08.30; to achieve this the whole team must assemble no later than 08.00, that time will be written into their contract so, if anyone is regularly late, they are guilty of fraud against the NHS. Anyone working in theatres could identify the culprits and I have watched it all my professional life; it is very rarely punished, usually only if management want to "get" the culprit for other reasons.

It should come as no surprise to anyone who has read this far that I have never known it happen where a team has been allowed to establish itself, but management are scared of teams. I have seen, not infrequently, an anaesthetist and a surgeon who detest each other (occasionally to the point where they would only communicate through a third party), work together very efficiently for many years. Each sufficiently respected the others shared specialist clinical abilities and commitment, to feel that any awkwardness, was worth tolerating for the provision of an excellent clinical service. It is, of course, preferable for everybody if one has a liking for a colleague whose abilities are such that they are a vital part of the team.

Perhaps this is an example of behaviour that justifies the management belief that doctors are unmanageable. But the consequence is that the clinical majority, finding that their own job plan is becoming increasingly unpleasant and restrictive, do really resent finding that some people are getting away with ignoring their job plan completely. If their wish to provide an efficient clinical service is also being blocked by the lazy and the cheats, then they, in turn, will either become disillusioned and lazy or will leave to find somewhere where a good efficient service is rewarded, not effectively punished; that is, pretty much, anywhere but the NHS.

It must be wrong to provide an extra incentive for someone simply to fulfil their contract, so this is a situation that calls for the stick not the carrot. Perhaps a bit of carrot would be a good idea for those clearly providing a clinical service above and beyond their contractual obligations. Once again, the difficulty for management in this is getting a handle on the metrics and the outcomes. In Chapter 11 I will suggest a radical, but cost neutral, restructuring of the NHS, a secondary benefit of which would be to make those metrics and outcomes much easier to obtain, and so enable the appropriate application of both the stick and the carrot.

This is a paradox where management difficulties are allowing a small proportion of doctors to cheat the system for their own advantage/comfort. The politicians seize on the situation as a justification for accusing all doctors of cheating the system, but, in fact, most doctors are vastly infuriated by it. Sometimes to the point where they just leave, either the NHS or the profession, or they retire early.

Sometimes the forces of inefficiency are truly insurmountable. Many years ago, at the very start of my specialised training, I worked in an elective orthopaedic hospital sited in a village about ten miles outside the city, where the main hospitals and all the other services were.

This was quite a common pattern; they were usually former tuberculosis sanatoria and it worked very well. The operating lists were scheduled to start at 08.30 and a newly appointed and enthusiastic consultant surgeon arrived on time for his list each week and would scrub and don his gown and gloves ready to start on time. He would then stand, in splendid isolation, in the middle of the theatre for about 20 minutes, becoming increasingly angry until he tore of his gloves and went to the phone to try and find out where everyone was. I was only there for a short time, so I do not know how long it took him to realise that the bus bringing the theatre nurses from the nurses' home in the city did not arrive until nine o'clock.

Most doctors in The NHS are general practitioners. It has always been my belief, although I have no particular evidence for it, that one of the prime motivations in founding the NHS was to ensure that everybody had good access to a GP. That is, free if payment would have been a deterrent and the opportunity to establish a relationship of continuing clinical care, for a family or community, with a reliable and nationally recognised doctor. If that was the idea, then it has become mangled, somewhere along the line, by the politico-bureaucratic machine that the NHS has become.

So far, I have written almost exclusively about hospital practice because that is whence my experience and insights into the NHS are derived; also, because this is intended as nothing more, or less, than a personal opinion. I must now confess that I know nothing of the frustrations or rewards of general practice, only a bit about the difficulties of continuity of care which have now arisen between GP's and hospital specialists.

I have spoken to one or two friends in general practice but have decided not to canvas thoughts widely from GP's, partly because I am sensible to the confusion consequent upon combining varying opinions; remember the definition of a camel as "a horse designed by a committee".

So, this remains a personal opinion, my apologies to any GP's who think that it is nonsense.

It is my impression that, as with hospital doctors, the general practitioners have become increasingly unhappy with their working environment over the last twenty to thirty years. At one time the salary was probably significantly less than for consultant specialists, although they did not have to undertake such a long period of training on a low salary. In the 1980's junior doctors pay was increased; I think that at around that time GPs' salaries were also brought more into line with hospital consultants. Later again, I think, under the intrusive New Labour Government, GPs were "given" the option of opting out of "out of hours on call" commitments. I suspect that the "option" was a theoretical one rather than a genuine choice, but, for whatever reason, they virtually all chose to take it.

Perhaps that was the beginning of the "family doctors" losing their role and their influence within the communities they served. I do not suppose the out of hours duties were particularly arduous, a small group or single person practice could arrange to share the rota with a neighbouring practice in the same community and most groups were large enough for the workload to be comfortable. What they lost was that all important sense of teamwork and continuity of care. It is difficult, in some respects impossible, certainly very time wasting and inefficient, to try and take on the care (safely) of another doctor's patient. In the old system, when called out to see a patient, they either knew them and their medical history, or they had easy access to notes, or could discuss them with their principal carer the next working morning, without having to spend hours on the telephone trying to track down a doctor they did not know.

For the trouble of going out at night or over a weekend everybody, patient, patient's family, on call doctor and regular GP, was happy that the problem had been dealt with as appropriately and safely as possible; and the doctors were very much appreciated in their community.

In its place a system was contrived which was, at least initially, organised by the GPs but which was completely impersonal and covered a far wider area than a couple of adjoining communities. As I understood it a syndicate of GPs ran an on-call system; some of them taking calls from patients and either giving advice, which might be to go to an A & E Department, or despatching a colleague on a home visit, if appropriate; some were those colleagues, in cars, doing the home visits as directed. The service was co-ordinated and provided by experienced GPs but lacked the ease of communication and continuity of care of the old long-established system.

I imagine it was imposed because it required fewer contracted on-call hours to pay GPs and therefore was cheaper, but at the cost of quality of care and patient safety.

Remembering that, despite their mantra, patient safety is not as important to managers and strategists as cost effectiveness, it is no surprise that the next step along the downward path was to out-source the service to agencies who under-cut the GPs bid, presumably by under-staffing the service. The next step appears to have been the realisation that it would be even cheaper if the people answering the phones were not doctors at all and there were no doctors available in cars to direct on house calls.

Welcome to the NHS 111 Phone Service!

Given the qualifications and experience of the people manning the phone lines it is probably right that the only advice they can give is "get yourself to the nearest A & E department". The A & E will be hopelessly over-run but that is the finance problem of the Hospital Trust, not the Community Services.

Not very joined up thinking for a supposedly National service.

More recently another scourge was introduced which must, I think, be very irritating for the GPs. In an effort to ration hospital care, without having to admit that that is the intention, a system was imposed whereby a GP could no longer refer a patient direct to a hospital specialist. They could only refer to what was called "a hub" clinic which was staffed by therapists and nurses, very able people on the whole with good clinical judgement, but they were under strict and monitored instructions to exhaust all forms of treatment before referring on for a specialist opinion, usually for some form of elective surgery. The patients were put through a time-consuming series of medical or physical programmes, which definitely reduced the rate of specialist referrals, but which rarely addressed the underlying physical problem in any lastingly useful or long-term way. This was hailed as a triumph by the managers and strategists, but it was only introducing a delay between onset of symptoms and optimal treatment, without having to use the politically unacceptable term of "waiting list".

It was also emasculating the GPs, whose role, prior to this introduction of another tier of expensive clinicians, was to judge the timing of when it was appropriate to refer a patient for, at least, a discussion about elective surgical options, if not an actual operation just yet. In my experience they were extremely good at it; I hardly ever received an inappropriate referral, whereas with the new system I often did not see patients until they had suffered an unnecessary and occasionally damaging delay.

The whole mess was then compounded by the introduction of a system which I can only imagine was dreamed up by some IT nerd, with little or no clinical background. It assumed that the entire population of the nation had easy access to and understanding of the internet. It was called "Choose and Book". On referral by a GP a patient would, soon afterwards, receive a letter containing a leaflet and about five typed pages giving them a "Booking Reference Number" and inviting them to choose between a number of clinics at which they could, by going online, book an appointment for themselves. A telephone number was given if they had any questions or could not get through online. This was pushed as giving the patient more control over their clinical destiny, but really, I suspect, it was just a way of ensuring that the referral had been approved (financially) by the relevant Care Provider. It also gives the providers the ability to control which unit gets the referrals, which they may well, in their target driven professional role, have a financial or political motivation to influence; certainly, it would not be a clinical reason.

I recently asked for a referral concerning a minor orthosis which I thought might be of benefit to me. I sat with my excellent GP while he made the referral (online) specifically naming the unit which I wished to attend. My letter duly arrived, with a Booking Reference Number, inviting me to choose between nine different units, for none of which I had any personal knowledge and many of which, by reputation, I would never attend under any circumstances; but not including the one unit I knew, which also happened to be the nearest. I called the number to ask if I could change to the unit of my choice and was told, by a booking clerk, that I could not because it had not been named by the GP, which I knew was not true.

I gave up.

Freedom of choice can, of course, only be meaningfully based on freedom of information. All the patient wants is for the GP to refer them to an appropriate specialist; there is no way that an individual can gather the information required to make an informed choice, because there is no way that the NHS can provide every patient with information that is useful and meaningful to them for every clinical contingency. But the GPs can and did make that judgement for them, very well, albeit with, perhaps, an inevitable bit of personal bias occasionally. Personal bias is not necessarily a bad thing, if a GP and a specialist know each other and get on well they are more likely to work together in the best interests of the patient. The chance to do that, professionally rather than just socially, has been blocked by the politicians.

These are all changes imposed on the GPs which I am aware of because they impinge on their relationship with the hospital services; important, but by no means their only, or even principal, role. I believe there must be many other things that the GPs are finding increasingly frustrating. Once again political targets have become an intrusive problem, this time linked with bribery, but still based on the obsession with management control. Many of the routine health checks, that the conscientious practices were performing already, were listed as obligatory tasks for which payment would be made. Things like the proportion of patients over a certain age having their blood pressure checked, the number having flu vaccinations and various other clinical assessments were subjected to performance assessments; but all it really achieved was to create another mountain of bureaucratic paperwork. This is reviewing quantifiable hard outcomes, but so much of a family doctors' vital work is about the unquantifiable soft outcomes, like spending time with patients who need it, for whatever reason. More paperwork that must result in less of the human touch.

Public expectations have also become quite unrealistic, sometimes even litigious; the "I know my rights and I will seek retribution for anything that I think infringes them" syndrome. Nothing could be more calculated to erode the patience, sympathy and commitment of a doctor trying to care for a community as best they can. It certainly does not inspire the doctor to work even harder but does have several unforeseen consequences. For instance, within a group practice there would often be a couple of partners who enjoyed performing minor operations under local anaesthetic; things like removal of small clinically benign lumps or stitching superficial lacerations. There is a miniscule risk that a lump might not be benign (that risk exists wherever and whoever removes it) or the wound might get infected (probably more of a risk in an A & E department) and they would probably have to take out extra indemnity against negligence claims. I believe they do have to take out indemnity if they do any out of hours work.

So, everybody is sent to the nightmare that A & E departments have become, because the GPs have had to abandon useful work that they enjoyed and was to everybody's benefit. They almost certainly did it a lot better than a stressed-out junior casualty doctor; nobody enjoys work they are not good at.

I think it must also be, at least in part, why young GPs are not interested in buying into a practice as a partner. That involves committing to a community and it is probably easier and just as well paid to work as an associate or even through an agency, allowing mobility, but at the cost of the fulfilment of caring and service. The patient load is too stressful, partly because there is nothing fulfilling about serving people who just want to make trouble. This is more likely in a transient urban community than a rural one, but wherever they work there are simply too few doctors for the UK population.

The GPs are the vital "gate-keepers" of The NHS and their prestige and morale have been remorselessly undermined by ill-judged political dicta over the last thirty years. They are the framework around which any good health care delivery system should be built. In virtually every country other than the UK anybody can self-refer to any "specialist" they wish to, whether they need a specialist opinion or not. As long as they can pay! That is a gross inefficiency. A well-functioning health service needs filters and that is a large part of the role which a doctor going into general practice wants to take on. They are particularly good at it, if they are allowed to get on with it; we do not need expensive extra filters whose sole function is to ration health care in a cheating and clandestine way. The GPs would not do that, so the politicians chose to bypass them, instead of tackling the underlying problem of demand being greater than supply.

If the NHS is to survive, let alone progress, through the 21st century then the GPs must be re-empowered and re-enthused to make their enormous contribution, probably the central theme of Bevan's concept in 1945, to the UK's unique health care delivery system.

Never having been a GP, I do not know precisely how that could best be achieved, but no doubt their Royal College would have some good ideas; it is time the politicians started listening.

Chapter 10

Private Compared to Public Health Care Delivery

In clinical medicine and surgery there is a relatively high demand for private care in some specialities and a low demand in others. Even within a single speciality there are variations. It is relatively high, for instance, in sports surgery or medicine and in arthritis surgery, but relatively low in children's orthopaedic surgery and trauma surgery. In specialist medicine it is relatively high in cardiology, particularly interventional cardiology, and relatively low in paediatrics or oncology. These variations partly reflect the differences in supply and demand which reflects the relative degree of urgency which the NHS, as a whole, assigns to different clinical conditions. It is, of course, entirely appropriate that children's afflictions, injuries and cancers should be high on that list.

It is also a reflection of the demographics of the different patient groups. Many people who require some form of treatment for arthritis can afford to pay for it and choose the flexibility of a time scale to suit them. Most parents who have a child born with a club foot or a congenital heart malformation are unlikely to be able to afford private treatment, but happily there is no reason why they should. Indeed, as I will go on to discuss later, there are many good reasons why they should not.

I like to think that, amongst all the reasons for choosing a particular speciality, the proportion of potential private practice is generally given the least consideration by most junior doctors choosing a training program. There are, of course, some for whom it is their chief consideration; although they may have a financially successful career, I hope they do not find it entirely fulfilling.

Whatever the reason, there will always be patients who wish to be treated privately and any healthcare delivery service should accommodate that wish. The reason for this is illustrated by the decision of the Canadian government to ban all private practice in their country. Waiting times for elective surgical procedures have steadily increased and there is a growing backlog of qualified trainees seeking consultant posts which no longer exist because their tenured aging occupants do not wish, or cannot afford, to retire. All that happens is that an increasing number of patients take themselves across the border into the USA for private treatment. If private treatment was not available in the United Kingdom, I have no doubt that exactly the same pattern would evolve, with patients taking themselves to continental Europe for treatment privately. That already occurs to some extent, with The NHS having to pick up the consequences of any complications. Since the demand is there, it should be met, the question is simply how best to do that in the interests of our own society.

The important question to consider about private practice is precisely why people wish to take up that option. I do not doubt that different people have various reasons, but probably the single most common one is the bizarre misconception amongst the UK population that private treatment is in some way superior to the state provision. My own belief is that within "western" society people value most highly those things that have cost them money; the more of an expensive rip off the better, it gives them a sense of ownership and of their own importance.

Probably, in about 90% of clinical situations exactly the opposite is true, the cases where private treatment is truly better, let alone safer, are, in fact, exceedingly rare.

This also manifests itself in the belief that certain treatments are only available privately because the NHS will always "choose" the cheapest rather than the "best" option. A good example of this is in the use of surgical implants. For instance, the choice of devices for joint replacement is vast. In general, those most recently developed by the manufacturing companies are the most expensive and the cheapest that are available are those that have been around for a long time; their development costs have long since been repaid and any patents will have expired. Many so-called technical improvements are based on theory and in the early years they can have no claim to have been proven in long term clinical practice. Quite often theoretical improvements turn out, in the fullness of time, to be exactly the opposite and some have been point-blank catastrophes, but the manufacturing companies will market their latest "improved" version very aggressively. These days this marketing is not confined to the orthopaedic surgical community, it is available to the general public through information technology and search engines. It is extremely plausible and convincing, sufficiently so not only to convince people with no inside knowledge of the subject, but also many (often recently appointed) practitioners within the orthopaedic community. Surgery, like everything else, is subject to fashion and a newly launched device can become very fashionable and extremely popular very quickly. It will, inevitably, have no long-term clinical outcome studies to justify its use but the mass media will jump on the bandwagon, proclaiming a new device as a triumphant breakthrough. This can be very misleading.

Around twenty years ago articles were appearing in praise of a particular type of hip replacement. I recall one with the headline "I'll never need a hip replacement; my hips are made of steel". That particular article included a background resume from a supposedly informed clinician; but one would think that any tabloid journalist must realise that anything the patient was not born with has to be some kind of replacement.

As the procedure became more widely adopted throughout the world, including by myself, unexpected problems emerged. Those scientists and surgeons who began to characterise the problems and identify risk factors for them, were initially ridiculed. But around ten years ago headlines started changing to things along the lines of "Toxic hip replacement has destroyed my life".

The truth, not surprisingly, lies somewhere between these two extremes. The devise is still in use and has excellent outcomes when chosen for the correct indications. There have been many instances of this type of situation with the introduction of a modified device, but if it attains a position of rapidly increasing popularity within the general public, before there is any experience of anything but short-term widespread usage, it is often only available in the private sector. The NHS, with a greater sense of its responsibilities to the public and less immediate interest in profitability, is prepared to hold back and wait to see what emerges in the longer term.

It is difficult and time consuming to give a fair and informative specialist consultation to a patient who opens proceedings by telling a surgeon that they want a particular type of joint replacement performed through a particular surgical approach. The first question that needs to be addressed is, "is a joint replacement the best treatment option for me in my current clinical situation"? If so, "what are the joint replacement options and what are the surgical approaches that might be optimal for me in the hands of you, as the surgeon"? Once an operation has been performed it can be modified or re-done (revised), but it can never be perfectly "un-done". The consultation is about ensuring that both the patient (including their family, if appropriate) and the surgical team are confident that it is the best option for a given clinical problem. It may be a less than perfect compromise; clinical therapeutic options are very rarely perfect!

If the surgeon and the patient find that they cannot reach any agreement the patient is free to seek a second opinion. Indeed, the surgeon himself should suggest that and make an agreed onward referral. This, of course, is easier and quicker to arrange for a private consultation, but it is definitely possible for an NHS one. Sadly, I have a distinct impression that with a private patient the initial consultant is more likely to just agree to perform the first demand, even if it is not something with which they are particularly familiar.

It can be quite dangerous being a private patient!

A medical equivalent of this is the preliminary publication of data without waiting for peer review. This has occurred recently with regard to Covid 19, it is often quite innocent in terms of the scientific team involved, but if it makes for a good headline, it will be conveyed in the mass media as though it were an established fact. Some years ago, this happened in a particularly unfortunate way which was definitely not "scientifically" innocent; the claim that Triple Vaccine against mumps, measles and rubella for children was linked with cases of Autistic Behaviour.

In this country the National Health Service avoided the mistake of giving these vaccinations separately, at greatly increased cost, but until it was established, beyond any possible doubt, that there was no basis of truth in the allegations a lot of parents denied their children the benefits of this very important and entirely safe immunity; with consequences that are still emerging.

A lot of other parents, only a little less foolish, sought private treatment for their children where charlatans were making a great deal of money by offering separate vaccinations at great expense and conferring no benefit.

I wonder if the coronavirus pandemic will finally establish in people's minds that a tried and trusted vaccine is an incredibly powerful and useful weapon in fighting crippling or life-threatening diseases? It seems not. You can convince all of the people some of the time and some of the people all of the time, but there will always be unbelievers. In general, most would agree that profoundly antisocial behaviour should carry some retribution; perhaps that should apply to a refusal to accept an established, proven effective and safe vaccination which is an important weapon in the eradication of a disease which is a danger to society at large.

Also, if you want the vaccination, do not pay for a "quick one" from a rogue supplier, wait until it is available on the National Health Service in the United Kingdom. This, happily, is what has mainly happened.

It can be not only dangerous, but also pointlessly expensive, being a private patient!

Another major misconception that is widespread among the general public is the question of whether private hospitals are preferable in every way, or even in any way, to state hospitals.

In this question, comparison of infection rates could be a useful guide. Despite many state hospitals having to function in overcrowded Victorian facilities, infection control is generally much better within the NHS than it is in the private sector. There are many reasons for this, but, in simple terms, in the former there is the possibility of using the advantages of multidisciplinary teamwork (admittedly not always made the best use of) and in the latter there is the inevitability of costs being minimised to maximise profits (almost always the overriding consideration).

In the public sector, so called, Hospital Acquired Infection Rates are rigorously examined and published. In the private sector everything from collecting the data to making it available seems rather more vague, so direct comparisons are not really possible.

It is my personal, clear impression that infection is a greater risk in the private sector; the difference in sterilising re-useable theatre instruments is a good example. In the NHS hospital I worked at there was a specialist Theatre Sterile Supply Unit (TSSU) within the theatre complex. Many orthopaedic instruments are modular, possibly also involving moving parts. These need to be disassembled, by someone who understands them, to be properly washed before being reassembled correctly, packaged in a sealed fashion and sterilised with marker tape which changes colour to show that the sterilisation cycle has been completed. Other trays have 30 or more different instruments or trial components in the tray. In our on-site specialist unit, the expert and well supervised staff knew what was meant to be on each tray and checked to make sure that nothing was missing, both when a used tray came out of a theatre, after the operation was completed and when the tray was re-packed ready for sterilisation; the theatre nurses knew to get the tray to TSSU as soon as the operation was completed. Some of the tools on these trays are very small, such as pins to hold a cutting block onto a bone. It is easy to lose one in a surgical site or amongst all the other instruments on the side tables, there might be 8 such pins on a given tray. The scrub nurse counts the contents of the tray as soon as it is agreed that it has served its purpose for that part of the operation. The golf ball has been played into the tree and that count is the first check to stop it emerging, but it is easy to count 7 as 8, especially with a grumpy surgeon who is not quite sure what he is trying to do (it happens when you are not in a familiar routine), is a bit scared and is venting his anxiety on the scrub nurse (which also, I am sad to say, happens not infrequently). The second count, in the rather calmer environment of TSSU, is a second check, done while the patient is still in the operating theatre complex and making doubly sure that the golf ball does not get through the tree.

None of this was possible in the private theatres because the scrub staff were not in a routine of orthopaedic procedures and had no idea what was meant to be on the tray, even if they understood the importance of checking it; so no first check. Then the trays, when they were finished with were not counted again by the scrub nurse, because they had no idea what was supposed to be in there anyway; so no second check.

The used trays were just put into a container to await a lorry coming to collect them, at the end of the day, to transfer them to a non-specialist TSSU 30 miles away, where nobody had a clue what they were used for, or whether they were modular and should be taken apart to be washed. No check three, the golf ball is still shooting through the tree and the presence of the pin deep in the wound is not revealed until the post-operative routine check X ray, and then only provided it is not obscured in both views by the metal of an implant.

There is another clear advantage to having an on-site specialist TSSU and that is that there could always be a store of sterilised instruments for various procedures available. Sometimes the sterilisation process fails; the packaging might have been damaged or there might be retained moisture inside the packaging which is not revealed until it is opened. Both these eventualities mean that the sterility of the contents cannot be guaranteed, but if it happens another pack can be opened in seconds. If another pack can only be sent from 30 miles away, in the middle of rush hour, the surgeon is faced with an unpleasant compromise choice. The operation can proceed with potentially unsterile instruments or there can be a delay of at least an hour with the patient anaesthetised on the table, a clear risk of an increase in the morbidity and mortality rates.

Another compromise on sterility is when instruments are introduced into the operating field which then transpire to have not been disassembled to be properly washed. This may reveal itself if they will not work properly or are jammed when they are supposed to be mobile, this did happen, not infrequently and one wonders how often it was the case without ever being apparent.

Also, not infrequently, trays would be found to be incomplete; not surprising given that they were not routinely checked. This may create a dilemma for the surgeon where they have to make cuts without the precise guides or choose a size that they do not feel is optimal. These compromises can be made, and the more familiar the surgeon is with the procedure the less impact they are likely to have, but it can jeopardise both the functional outcome and the long-term survival of an implant. They also, indirectly, increase the risk of infection as that rises the longer an operation takes and the more people there are entering and leaving the theatre.

Where would you rather have your operation for, for instance, a joint replacement?

The advantages, in orthopaedics at least, in having an on-site specialist TSSU are manifest, but a service of sorts can be provided more cheaply. There were repeated suggestions from management that our TSSU should be closed as a service could be provided more "efficiently" from an off-site combined unit. Efficient, of course, is management new-speak for a cost saving at the expense of patient well-being and safety; there will be much posturing about equality and "level playing fields". It is easy to justify a non-specialist unit not needing a specialist TSSU, but to extrapolate that to a specialist unit is absurd.

It is like stating that, because some playing fields are mud patches strewn with litter including broken bottles and used needles, all playing fields should be like that. Not everybody can have access to the lush turf of Twickenham, so nobody should have it. The cry of justice and equality, once again, driving everybody to the lowest common denominator.

So far, the surgeons have resisted these plans, but unless something changes, sooner or later they will lose their specialist TSSU.

Continuity of care is an important concept where the private hospitals can fail dreadfully. I have written about this concept and its overwhelming importance in an earlier chapter. In a private operating theatre, a surgeon is very unlikely to see the same team twice running. On the wards the patients are unlikely to see the same nursing staff twice, let alone consecutively over two days.

The resident medical officers are covering, in all probability, a vast number of different consultant clinicians with no insight into what each one feels is important or might be concerned about. A few surgeons make sure that they only operate with somebody they know and trust as an assistant, but many do not. I personally, for instance, would only operate in a private hospital if accompanied by a very experienced senior theatre sister from my NHS hospital. She was not only the best assistant I could have but could also watch the theatre scrub team to make sure they were not about to do anything inappropriate and, as very frequently happened, stop them before it caused any problems.

This lack of any recognisable clinical team leaves consultant clinicians very exposed working in a private hospital. For any but the most obsessive personalities it is simply not possible to be available, on call, for twenty-four hours a day seven days a week.

I have often wondered how a single obstetrician can adequately provide private cover for the delivery of a baby. It may be reasonable for a surgeon to offer a patient a private elective operation at a time that suits them when the surgeon can make himself available for the necessary length of time. It is appropriate for a cardiologist to give a private consultation and opinion to a patient, but it would not be for him to take a fee agreeing to be available as a matter of urgency if that patient suffers a heart attack. With obstetrics it simply cannot be done to cover an event which may happen at any time over about a six-week period, like the birth, or complications in the birth, of an infant. Yet private obstetric services are on offer; anecdotally, it seems to me that most obstetric problems, or even disasters, arise when the private consultant cannot be found and other junior staff are reluctant to step in, without the consultant's permission.

Just as the consultant clinician working in the private sector has little in the way of a support team, it follows that there is little in the way of peer review or regulation.

In the public sector there is a mandatory obligation to undertake, together with all the other consultants in the group providing the same or a related specialist service, a regular meeting known as a Morbidity and Mortality Review. Most groups do this every one or two months and each clinician's clinical work for that period is presented, usually by one of the trainees, and all unexpected outcomes or complications are discussed by the individual's peers. Morbidity is a less than optimal event and mortality is the ultimate hard outcome; could, or should, anything have been done differently? Usually, the result of the discussion is that the complication was unavoidable and that there was nothing inappropriate in the selected treatment or the way in which it was undertaken but remember that doctors are like manure; these meetings are certainly no cover-up exercise. It is a fantastic way of teaching, learning and sharing experience and it does not take long to identify if an individual is practicing in some way outside the accepted parameters. That very rarely occurs because things are open and under review.

Of all the meetings I had to attend these were the ones I found the most useful, productive and enjoyable.

I imagine that some consultants, perhaps if most of their work is in the private sector, do conduct some kind of peer review with colleagues concerning their private clinical outcomes, but I never succeeded in persuading my group to include their private patients in our regular reviews. Possibly because we would have had to collate the data ourselves instead of having a trainee to do it, but consultants are, inappropriately, very secretive about their private practice. The fact is that if any consultant working in a private hospital does not want to have his work reviewed by his peers there is no obligation for him to do so. Some consultants, quite simply, cheat on their patients.

One form of cheating is to undertake procedures or investigations that simply do not need to be done. This happens, particularly with unnecessary investigations, but is probably quite rare; there is no data regarding these practices as nothing is properly regulated. Another, more subtle way, of misleading a patient is, I have no doubt, quite commonly perpetrated. That is to undertake a procedure that is not truly within the clinician's field of special interest or expertise.

There is abundant evidence that specialists who undertake a given procedure regularly and, within the confines of the frequency of the clinical problem, often, will consistently achieve better outcomes than people who do the same procedure relatively rarely. This is really not surprising and put simply it means that there is no place for somebody to do something once every six months when they have a colleague in the next-door clinic who does it six times a week.

It is not uncommon for surgeons in private hospitals to undertake procedures on private patients which they do not perform, or offer, for the National Health Service.

Sometimes they are even aided and abetted in this by the private hospital itself. Patients sometimes enquire of a private hospital whom they have practicing with them who can perform a given procedure, shall we say a hip replacement? I have known one hospital, at least, which would give out the name and contact details to the enquirer of two spinal surgeons and a trauma surgeon, none of whom ever did hip replacements on the NHS. Yet there were other surgeons in that hospital whose particular NHS interest was hip replacement surgery. I do not think this is anything more sinister than just another example of the complete lack of insight and regulation which exists in the private sector; but then, I think that is pretty sinister in itself.

Rarely it happens in a more sinister and damaging way. For instance, a surgeon who has the inclination to undertake questionable, or possibly unnecessary, procedures on patients will be much more likely to do so in a private hospital, where he is not subject to observation by other colleagues or at any risk of peer review such as regular morbidity and mortality meetings. A breast surgeon was recently convicted, and imprisoned, for performing multiple unnecessary operations on many women, primarily by telling them that they had some type of cancer. Most of the operations were carried out in a private hospital, either on private patients or on NHS patients who had been sold off into the private sector under the appalling choose and book scheme. He should have been caught much sooner; he would have been in an NHS hospital.

These are all hazards for patients, or weaknesses, in private healthcare delivery in this country, but there is one aspect of private health care provision which is, in my opinion, particularly malign and misleading – that is private health insurance. All insurance companies are profit making organisations. They have to be, because otherwise they could not make any payments, nobody would take out insurance with them. The companies make their profits by following the advice of actuaries. An actuary is a mathematician who analyses statistics to calculate the insurance risk premiums. The word derives from the Latin *actuarius* which means bookkeeper. Insurance companies are, in fact, just bookies who are analysing the odds to ensure that they make a profit.

Some forms of insurance are obviously sensible, for instance, life insurance. Other forms of insurance are obligatory, either legally, like motor insurance for driving, or financially like home insurance for securing a mortgage; but no resident of the United Kingdom has any need whatsoever for healthcare insurance (except for travel outside the UK) because the state provides that free at the time of need. I call healthcare insurers malignant because of the deceitful way in which they market and advertise their product.

Superficially health care insurance seems no different from any other form of insurance. The sales pitch is logical and persuasive, you can choose from different companies on comparison sites, you can customise the package to suit your personal requirements and you can change the precise details if your circumstances change. But they have, effectively, a "captive audience" because only the reasonably affluent middle classes, or those who are even richer, can afford the insurance or are interested in it. There are two very important differences which, in practice, are only revealed by taking out the insurance and then living with it into old age. First, the annual premium will inevitably and inexorably increase with the passage of time, the number of exclusions is also likely to increase. Second, the premium is very low during a lifetime phase when people are unlikely to have a medical problem and make a claim. As the cost begins to rise rapidly the fact that you did not need the insurance in the first place has a paradoxical effect; realising that they have already spent a lot for nothing people are reluctant to admit that money was a total waste and fall into the ongoing trap of throwing good money after bad.

This information is all available, but people just do not seem to realise its significance until it is too late. As a provider for patients who are insured it becomes increasingly obvious the more one talks to them. The package works like this. They trap young families with apparently generously low premiums to include children (a very emotive issue which would be tempting to all parents). Often the private health insurance is included as part of the financial package of a salary. People, not surprisingly, fall into this trap but in actuarial terms a young family is extremely unlikely to incur any significant medical expenses as a private patient. The "victim" probably realises that, but the fear of some ghastly accident or catastrophic medical disaster occurring to one of their children remains. It is a potent motivator. Once the children are past adolescence, just as they enter, actuarially, the highest risk age range for serious accidents, unless they are still living in the parental household, they are no longer considered part of the family and therefore no longer insured. The parents however continue paying the premiums and maintaining their insurance. If it ceases to be part of their salary package, or it never was, they are probably affluent enough to pay it anyway because the premiums remain pretty low. That is, until they reach the age of 60 when they are just entering, actuarially, the time when they are most likely to incur medical fees as a private patient. At that point the cost escalates rapidly, but by then the victim feels locked into the treadmill. The premium is something that is factored into their background expenses and even if their spending power is diminished, having retired, it takes quite a dramatic and radical rethink to factor it out.

There are other reasons why I describe this financial package as misleading. It advertises on the basis that it enables you to see a specialist of your choice quickly and easily in pleasant surroundings, but that is by no means certain to be the case. A consultation fee with a doctor should not be particularly expensive and for any kind of treatment the doctor's fee is usually a relatively small part of the total bill. However, like any successful business, the insurance companies are constantly looking for ways of reducing costs in order to maximise profits and the easiest thing to drive down is not the hospital costs (they often own and run the hospitals themselves anyway), but the doctors' fees.

To this end they have created a system whereby specialists have to sign on with the insurance company, accepting the excessively low fees that they impose. If they do not agree to this, then the company will not recommend them. It is exceedingly difficult for a potential patient to gather information about which consultant might be the best person to see regarding their particular symptoms and condition. In the old days one could rely on the GPs, but the ridiculous choose and book appointment system has rather blown away the chances of a GP and specialist forming a working familiarity and trust with each other, teamwork again.

Recommendations often go by word of mouth around a community, a village, social club, sports club, etc but that is not always particularly reliable. I can think of many specialists whom I would be happy to socialise with but would not let make any decision about the management of a condition, let alone implement its treatment. Established specialists can and do build their reputation within their community, but that can be undermined by one unlucky and very disgruntled patient. Probably the most reliable way of choosing a specialist for any given condition is to find out if they treat many patients with that condition on the NHS, because it is their principal interest. Even armed with this information the insured patient may find that the specialist of their choice was not prepared to drop their long-established fees in order to enlarge the profits of the insurance company.

In that situation the honourable thing for the insurance company to do would be to accept that the patient has the right to see whom they choose (as, in theory, all NHS patients have), but to warn them that there will be a shortfall between the specialist's fees and what they are prepared to reimburse; but that the vast majority, if not all, other treatment fees will be covered by the insurance. Surprise, surprise, that is not what they do. They simply inform the patient, their client, that they are not allowed to see the specialist of their choice and provide them with a list of specialists who are acceptable to them i.e., have signed up to their cartel. As I have already pointed out the named specialist that they accept may not even treat that condition at all on the NHS.

I have spent my professional lifetime trying to persuade my coterie of, mainly affluent and intelligent, friends that private health insurance is a waste of money. Their reply is usually something along the lines of "but what about the really serious illness that is going to be very expensive to treat". The answer to that is simple. Anyone who suffers a really serious long term or life-threatening illness is far better off being treated on the NHS anyway. Those sorts of conditions often require a multidisciplinary approach and inpatients in that situation must have a 24-hours a day seven days a week clinical team supervising their management. If there is a crisis in that type of condition for a private patient and the relevant consultant cannot be contacted, then any prospect of that vital continuity of care is likely to be blown away. It is much safer being treated as an NHS patient, where continuity of care, if not absolutely guaranteed, is at least a distinct probability.

For that reason alone, private health insurance is worse than just a waste of money, it is positively dangerous.

Here is another reason.

I was not long into my own consultant appointment before I recognised a consistent pattern that was, sadly, repeated over the thirty-plus years of my consultancy. I was appointed to work specifically and only in the specialised field of joint replacement, particularly attempting to correct joint replacements that had failed or gone wrong in some way. That does not guarantee that I necessarily became very good at it, but it is certainly the environment which gives anybody the best possible chance of being good at it.

It became obvious that patients with any kind of complicated surgical problem were being referred to me after two or three inappropriate and unsuccessful surgical attempts to correct it; if they had private health insurance. If they were NHS patients, they were usually referred immediately following a single NHS consultation about the problem.

Every operation that fails to correct a surgical problem diminishes the chances of any subsequent operation achieving this and increases the difficulty and extent of subsequent operations. It also worsens the eventual functional outcome. A successful first-time hip or knee replacement will function better than one that has already been revised once, let alone two or three times.

The perfect patient for such a joint replacement is one who is going to die before the joint replacement fails or wears out. That is, die many years later, from unrelated causes while the joint is still functioning well. The most likely way to achieve this is for the patient to be above the age of about 65 at the time of their initial surgery, but sometimes it is appropriate and necessary to do joint replacements on people in their twenties or thirties.

Such patients would be expected to live longer than the predictable working life of an artificial joint and will be facing one, or more revisions during their natural lifespan. If a complication like a fracture, or more especially, an infection around an implant occurs then they will require further surgery many years before it had been hoped. If two or three attempts at correcting this, with obvious technical imperfections ensuring further failure, are undertaken, then a patient in their thirties may find that they have the type of salvage implant, surrounded by the extensive muscle damage and scar tissue that is the inevitable consequence of three or four operations. But this has occurred over a period of two or three months, while they are still aged in their thirties, not over forty or fifty years, taking them into their eighties, as they could reasonably have hoped. This, of course, is accompanied by the kind of exceedingly poor functional outcome that might be acceptable to an eighty-year-old but is a terrible burden for someone in their thirties with young children.

The best chance to correct a surgical problem is with the first surgical attempt to do so.

The best chance to achieve this lies with a surgeon who is familiar with dealing with the problem.

The surest way to minimise the chance of being immediately referred to an appropriate surgeon is by having private health insurance.

A sad reflection on human nature, but irrefutably true.

Oscar Wilde said, with some cynicism but a lot of perspicacity, that "experience is the name we give to our mistakes". He could have added that a lot of experience can also be gained from other peoples' mistakes.

So, what of public health care delivery. The NHS is far from perfect and can certainly be improved. Indeed, it must evolve if it is to survive. I have given examples throughout this book of why I think that the NHS and public health care delivery is superior, in almost every important respect, to private health care delivery (which lies outside the routine controls and support of the NHS) and there is little point in repeating those. But there is one aspect of health care delivery, which is very highly valued by patients, in which the private sector almost invariably performs better than the NHS. That is access; the ease with which a patient can contact a relevant clinician to discuss a new concern or initiate a review of an existing one. The reason for this is easily understood, in the private sector access equates to income but in the NHS, it is seen as a drain on a limited resource. This is really just a misconception, an attitude on the part, primarily, of the management rather than the clinicians. There is no real reason why it should not be completely reversed with no cost implications.

The first vital step, as is so often the case, is access to the GPs, the best possible filters and gatekeepers of the NHS. All this really requires is standardisation. Many GP practices provide excellent access for patients. As I have said, I do not know why others seem unable to; but if it is possible for some groups, it should be possible for all. Then, the totally artificial restrictions of access to specialist opinions, imposed by management strategists, could be swept away: the "Choose and Book" referral system with its extra tier of therapists instructed to exhaust all non-operative treatments for conditions which inevitably will require a surgical solution (cataracts, hernias, arthritis, etc.); secretaries forbidden to take calls from patients already in a service but with a fresh concern; the rigid restrictions on internal referrals from one specialist service to another (a specialist referral that turns out to be inappropriate or that reveals a different clinical problem meaning that the patient has to make a completely fresh start with the ludicrous choose and book system). There are just dozens of little ways in which access for patients to a clinical service is made frustratingly and unnecessarily difficult.

So many of the important improvements in clinical care that must be achieved by the NHS do not require anything more than a change of attitude and established habits. There is often no need for seismic restructuring, expensive consultancy reviews, shifts in the balance of personnel or vastly increased expenditure.

I will conclude this comparison of private and public health care delivery systems by giving an example of what can result if an entire nation's health care delivery is dominated by unrestrained commercial forces.

Almost certainly the most dangerous aspect of private health care delivery is the lack of regulation and ongoing peer review. If the NHS is one of the best examples of a state-run service, then the most complete example of the opposite, in a comparable socio-economic western society, must be the USA. The USA has many fine and world respected University hospital structures in the major cities, but most of the health care to the population is delivered from an office-based practice. That is a small and relatively isolated group of doctors banding together to form a clinic, based on a small and relatively isolated hospital, in a relatively small town. We will look specifically at total hip replacement, a classic quality of life elective procedure which is common. It is generally ranked as the second most successful operation ever devised, with cataract surgery as the first because it is simpler to perform and carries fewer life-threatening risks.

A few years ago, it was widely accepted on the "international hip surgery conference circuit" (a generally useful source of information, although I sometimes think of it as the bullshit trail) that 70% of the hip replacements performed in the USA each year were done by surgeons who did less than seven cases per year. Nobody doubts that the surest way of becoming adept at a procedure is to do it fairly frequently and the only way, realistically, that you could fall into the hands of such an infrequent practitioner of a procedure in this country is if you were recommended/compelled by your private health insurance company, if you are foolish enough to have one, to consult one of those surgeons who undertakes operations privately that they do not offer at all on the NHS, part of their cartel, with no interest in patient welfare.

A figure called the Revision Burden is a mathematical way of expressing the number of revisions that would be generated within a community or nation as a percentage of the number of initial joint replacements. That is the risk of it failing expressed as a percentage and a measure of how long the initial replacement lasted. The revision of a joint replacement is at least four times, often many times, more expensive than the initial procedure. In general, the Scandinavian countries have the lowest revision burdens, but the UK is not far behind, whereas the USA has, close to, if not the highest revision burden in the world.

How can this be?

This is the richest and most powerful economy the world has ever seen, spending by far the highest proportion per capita of any country in the world on health care delivery. But, for its entire population, it is performing badly in comparison to other western economies in many respects (as discussed in Chapter 2), which include patient care provision and "satisfaction" as well as "value for expenditure".

Half its expenditure is in private provision and it is a Nation of extremes of wealth and poverty. Perhaps the half that is left for the poor just has to be spread very thinly; but I have never believed that to be a valid explanation. Much of the state provision of health care in the USA comes from the University Hospitals and The Veterans Administration System. These are extremely well equipped, well-staffed and well administered providers that cover a very large proportion of the population. In any case, hip replacement for end stage joint failure is a health care provision to a predominantly affluent section of society, which is why 70% of it is delivered privately through an office-based practice.

We should beware in the UK. There is no justification for smug complacency. In some respects, health care delivery is probably better regulated in The US than anywhere in the world; they were years ahead of us in things like continuing medical education and five yearly regulated revalidation of clinicians; but this is regulation of training and knowledge, not of judgement, experience, profit and expenditure.

There are many University and religious foundation teaching hospitals, mainly on the East and West Coasts which make huge contributions to our understanding of hip replacement. So why do they, as a nation, perform it so badly?

I believe it is the natural end point of un-restrained commercial pressures and greed, driven with no nation-wide overview or regulation. The value of The US market for orthopaedic implants is the same as the whole of the rest of the world put together and the number of different devises available is vast; each one with "champion surgeons" and a marketing team. A member of the marketing team is usually called in as a technical advisor for each one of the 7 office-based implantations per year. Their principal occupation is to advise on the technique for implanting that device, whereas the surgical team only see it once every 7 or 8 weeks. The cost of all this is large, as are the rewards for the manufacturer and the marketing and surgical teams.

In this situation each surgeon's choice of which particular hip replacement system to use is driven by commercial pressures and fashion. Not by peer review of long-term outcomes and Federal regulation. The opposite of the Scandinavian countries or our NHS, with the result that a vast array of unproven devises is implanted.

Furthermore, the whole charade is conducted against a background of high litigation risk and thus, high insurance costs.

Result, in a meaningful marker of performance with a hugely successful therapeutic intervention in a largely affluent population their costs are astronomical, with clinical results that are, point blank, appalling.

Is this the way forward for health care delivery in the UK? The NHS being sold off, piecemeal, to private profiteers. Some people think so, we must be incredibly careful. B movies and fast-food burgers may be almost intolerable, but at least they do not (directly) kill or maim you.

Chapter 11

Saving the NHS. A Possible Solution?

Much of what I have written this far seems to have come out as a castigation of private clinical practice; I did not expect it to be that way, but it seems that is how my thinking has evolved as I have written. I have no problem with the concept of private practice, indeed I should now stress, as I have stated earlier, that I believe it to be an important element in any health care delivery system. My concerns are about the poor, almost non-existent, regulation of private clinical practice, including the institutions in which it takes place and the corrupt activities that have grown up around it. But there will always be a demand for private treatment and if it is not available in this country patients will simply go elsewhere for it, as the Canadians do; much to the disadvantage of their own nation and often themselves.

If you have read this far, I hope that by now you believe, at least, that private health insurance for the inhabitants of the UK is a pernicious misrepresentation that has to be the worst financial deal in the marketplace since the South Sea Bubble two hundred years ago. It is just another middleman taking a cut from the overall cost of health delivery, sometimes in a destructive way, without contributing anything to the overall evaluation and improvement of heath care.

It should be banned.

You may also feel that it could be a good thing if clinicians practicing in the private sector were better regulated when doing so. If you do not, then you risk, perhaps unintentionally, supporting the expansion of poorly regulated private health care activity and the piecemeal dismantlement of the NHS. You may be tossing burning faggots onto Eden's Funeral Pyre.

So, can we reconcile the demand for private treatment with the need for it to be better regulated than it is anywhere else in the world, where there is also, effectively, little or no regulation? Perhaps we can.

Perhaps all private consultations and treatments should be delivered within the framework of the NHS, which is a potential advantage that we do have over every other nation. Every aspect of health care should be incorporated under the NHS umbrella. Every private hospital, private clinic, private rehabilitation centre, and private residential home in the country should be acquired by the NHS. It sounds like a mammoth undertaking, but there was something faintly obscene about The NHS having to pay private facilities for the use of beds in intensive care units during a national emergency; those same private facilities that had spent years profiteering at the expense of the NHS.

In any case, I suspect it would involve many fewer disruptive compulsory purchases than the HS2 rail project, currently going nowhere, at vast expense and doubtless ending up as another Millennium Dome white elephant. It is, after all, only bringing the project started by Bevan in 1945 to its logical conclusion. Just as for Bevan, it will require a government with a large majority that is prepared to disrupt some established, but outmoded, patterns. We currently have a government with a large majority, although at the time of going to press that seems to be in some jeopardy. If it survives let us see if they are capable of thinking outside the box.

This should be described as a "further incorporation", or some other term of political newspeak. It must not be referred to as a Nationalisation. That word is inescapably associated in too many peoples' minds (including mine) with political dogma, massive bureaucracy, poor service provision and ultimate catastrophic failure. But some public services, the military, the police, air traffic control, etc. are simply better under the care of The State. It would also open, potentially, a huge new funding stream; public funds, in a post-pandemic economy, are going to be tight.

One of the benefits of separating, within the NHS, the purchasing authorities from the providing Trusts is that the cost of every procedure undertaken had to be evaluated. This will always be an evolving estimate but at least we now have a reasonable idea of the cost, known as the tariff, of a given surgical procedure, investigation or medical treatment. The NHS should certainly continue to provide all appropriate medical and social care, free at "the time of need". The time of need is a much better term than "the point of delivery", as delivery may be unduly untimely. Even so, the time of need will be subject to variations according to other conflicting services and there will always continue to be some delay for treatment of conditions that are not life or limb threatening, largely elective surgery.

This creates a perfect situation for people to pay for their treatment if that is appropriate and they wish to. I learnt over the years that the doctor should not fall into the error of judging who can or cannot afford to pay for private treatment. It is one thing to inform a patient that they can be treated just as well on the NHS, sometimes better and comparably as quickly or even faster, as they can privately. As well or better, on the NHS is usually true. Sooner is quite often the case, much to the patient's surprise. But the doctor can have no knowledge of the patient's ability to pay, to appear to be withholding the option of private treatment, on purely financial grounds, is invading their privacy in a snobbish and patronising manner.

On the other hand, many people whom I treated privately expressed a feeling of guilt that they were in some way jumping the queue and cheating other NHS patients. This, of course, was a total misconception; an NHS contract includes a fixed amount of theatre time for operations and only NHS patients are treated on those lists. There is no facility to do more NHS lists and patients because there is no funding. But if the patient chose to pay the Purchasing Authority tariff themselves the providing trust could arrange lists in an NHS theatre, staffed by clinicians working on NHS time. The purchasing authority does not have the funds to run the theatre at that time, but this would enable the provider to run more NHS lists than the state purchaser can afford.

At present a patient who wishes to pay for their treatment must undertake to pay a fee for professional services, not an exorbitant sum, but must also pay for theatre usage, in-patient time and nursing, all therapist input, all disposables, all drugs and implants used, etc. That really does add up to a considerable sum of money; usually 6 to 8 times the combined fee for both the surgeon and anaesthetist, but still only about the same as a couple of years premiums for private health insurance for most people seeking, for instance, a hip replacement. Any private insurance company is also likely to impose clinical restrictions in order to maximise their profit.

Perhaps there should be the option for patients to pay the purchasing authority tariff themselves, a kind of voluntary, optional, self-evaluated means testing. Standard means testing is a laborious, inefficient and invasive procedure which is notoriously open to abuse and which, if applied rigorously, only penalises those who already pay the most tax. This treatment pathway could be presented as a way in which those who are able to would support the NHS, enabling it to treat more patients who really do require their treatment to be FREE at the time of need. Nobody need choose it if they did not wish to and therefore there needs to be some incentive beyond pure altruism.

That would be time. Those who choose the pathway should be given a provisional date for their treatment, with a significantly shorter waiting time and a named consultant, of their choice if they want, to supervise their treatment. Apart from the benefit of being (relatively) fast tracked they would, in every way, be an NHS patient. No promise of a private room, or that the consultant would perform the procedure personally, students and trainees involved in their care, involvement (if they agree) in clinical trials and, although they could plan for the timing of their treatment, nothing more than a strong probability that it would be completed on the provisional date.

The option should primarily be available for non-life or limb threatening conditions, which is what elective surgery is, but there are various medical conditions which would also fit logically into the group. The appropriate clinical conditions would be largely self-defining as they would be those for which there is already a significant delay in the NHS. Some might choose to follow that pathway anyway, especially if there was a further incentive such as making self-payment of tariff tax deductible.

Tax exempt or not, the cost to the patient would be a fraction of the cost of maintaining private health insurance for several years. The big administrative difficulty is that the scheme would have to be carefully (and impartially) monitored and reviewed to maintain a fair balance between the "fast track incentive" and delivery to others at "the time of need"; but that should be perfectly possible.

The patients would be referred by their GP to an appropriate NHS specialist service and seen by a consultant or another clinician working with that consultant. Sometimes a consultant will feel that there are good clinical or social reasons (domestic, as a carer for instance, or seasonal employment commitments) to time a planned treatment in advance, typically for an operation. Those patients could be given a specific date, which would not necessarily be the earliest available, with a strong probability that the treatment would go through on that day.

Most patients would be considered as routine and would simply be added to a list for treatment. Once listed, the patient would be seen by someone from administration to choose their track and complete the necessary details, including the financial commitments if they chose to be self-payers. If they were self-payers, they would be given a provisional date, if not they would be given an approximate time scale. The important thing is that when they come for their treatment no clinician need know which track they had chosen. They are all standard NHS patients.

The extra income, over and above what the purchasing authority could afford, would enable the provider trust to use its plant and staffing more fully and efficiently. The clinicians would not require additional payments as they are simply treating NHS patients within the framework of their job plan.

There would then be a third and final tier of access to health care, under the global umbrella of the NHS, which would embrace those patients who specifically wish to be a private patient in a private room and will take themselves overseas if that option does not exist in the UK. At current rates that, for most procedures, would cost about three times the tariff rate, still cheaper for most patients than maintaining private insurance. For that they would have a date of their choice (within reason), although still with no absolute assurance that that date could be fulfilled, an undertaking by the consultant of their choice (for what that is worth) to personally perform the procedure and all the other minor irrelevancies that are usually associated with being a private patient. The treatments are delivered by consultants outside the hours of their contracted NHS job plan and therefore the patient pays them a fee, but it is delivered in a properly regulated NHS hospital, which also charges a fee.

It is a bit like airline travel. You can choose to fly carriage class, business class or first class and there are greater or lesser advantages in each more expensive class, in terms of the pre-flight check in times and waiting area privacy. There are inflight advantages in terms of the level of comfort and there are some advantages in terms of the ease of disembarkation and passage through immigration and customs. The most significant difference is just the cost. All passengers have the same inflight delays before take-off, the same arrival time, the same inflight delays to arrival, whilst stacking over Heathrow for instance, the same risk of being blown out of the sky by an itinerant missile or flown into a hillside by a demented pilot or an overcomplicated computer system. It is a matter of individual choice.

In a three-tier NHS comparison the risks and benefits of the treatment or procedure planned are the same for everybody, the quality of clinical care is the same for everybody; there are, perhaps, the soft advantages of a greater degree of continuity of care and timing of care for the private patient, but otherwise it is entirely comparable. The idea of a three-tier system may be abhorrent to some bizarre individuals; I can hear the howls of indignation from the anarchic Marxists and the cacophony of violent protests. But total equality of outcome is not really achievable for humankind, except by inflicting the lowest common denominator on everyone. What any civilised society should be striving for is equality of opportunity. In this three-tier system everyone has the same opportunity to spend money if they wish to, to choose which pathway suits them best and to accept the same clinical risks whilst receiving pretty much identical clinical care under the same state system. No-one is profiteering or taking advantage of anyone and the fully private care is properly regulated and peer reviewed.

Equality!

There is a risk that it would simply be used as another excuse to introduce a huge new tier of managers, but there would really be no justification for that. Some aspects of hospital management would be easier; for instance, controlling the consultant clinicians. Every clinician's job plan is reviewed each year as part of their annual performance appraisal and each consultant could put in a bid for what proportion of private to public work they wished to undertake, based on the experience of the previous year's demand. Income from the private patients, who are paying more than the basic tariff, could be retained by the providing Trust giving them greater financial flexibility. My personal choice for the best use of this income, which previously went to the profiteers outside the NHS, would be to ensure that space was retained for staff facilities, as I mentioned in a previous chapter.

It would also provide the managers with the easily collected and irrefutable data, that they long for, to enable them to control the clinicians. They would know precisely what proportion of a consultant's time was being spent on the NHS patients (NHS tariff state paid and NHS tariff self-paid) and what proportion on private patients. If a consultant failed to fulfil his contractual obligation to the NHS, he could have his practicing rights for private patients suspended. I think that any sensible clinician would also like the arrangement because it is safely managing private patients in a health service hospital, with cover from junior staff and trainees; much less demanding than being isolated in a private hospital. Also, the NHS could pick up the litigation insurance for every patient treated on the trust site, probably at marginal extra cost as the "site" and its activities are well regulated. The clinicians would not then need to take out separate, and often frighteningly expensive, indemnity against litigation from private treatments in a high-risk environment.

I think this system could also work well for social care, all of which would be under The NHS umbrella. As Bevan, said when he combined being Minister of Housing with The Health Ministry, "all communities should be a microcosm of the society at large" and I can see this working in a care home. Some residents would pay nothing for their care, others would be able to, and might wish to, pay more; perhaps to have more space or a different diet. For all of them the actual care would be the same and they would represent a varied community from all sorts of social backgrounds. This is what happens for the undergraduates in the better of our universities.

I am not sure how it would work for the General Practitioners; I confess I have no personal insight into this. The only thing that I would suggest is that it should block those General Practitioners who only wish to see private patients. All GPs should offer some degree of NHS practice, although they could negotiate to have a low level if they felt that appropriate.

This seems to me to be a good, perhaps the best, way of getting rid of the profiteering and poorly regulated elements of private practice, whilst enriching the public sector and embracing a genuine concern for patient safety in all aspects of the Nation's health care delivery. Currently it is extremely difficult, probably impossible, to regulate private activity properly.

A frequent criticism of the NHS, including from myself, is poor management systems, but I believe that it would be easier to improve management patterns within the NHS than to change the private profiteers into public spirited organisations and individuals.

Chapter 12

The Future through Research and the Coronavirus Effect

I have previously written that the NHS must evolve if it is to survive and, for health care delivery, evolution must be based on research. It would be inappropriate to write about health care without acknowledging that progress can only be made as a result of research and the benefits have been dramatically highlighted through the recent pandemic, in many ways. But not all research projects lead to useful or beneficial results, as has been found many times in the field of joint replacements.

At its simplest, observation and deduction are a research project, but even that is fraught with risk of erroneous conclusions, particularly with the soft outcomes which are such a feature of health care. All research requires financial and workforce investment, the more complex and technologically demanding the greater the expense, but potentially also, the greater the benefits. This is the perfect field of endeavor for collaboration between the NHS clinical services, with their already established university links, and commercial enterprises. There are many examples of this pattern being extremely productive, the incredible production of covid 19 vaccines being the most obvious recent one.

In general, the key to successful development, progress, modernization – call it whatever – is just that it should be evolutionary; a gradual development that asserts itself because the benefits become manifest. Not something that is imposed from extraneous forces because of some transient philosophical dogma or new technological possibility. In the UK, the architecture of the 1960's and 70's is an example, with monstrous tower blocks and concrete jungles being imposed upon communities just because they had become a constructional possibility. The law of unforeseen consequences soon rendered them uninhabitable for any civilized society. Great care must be taken to ensure that these kinds of mistakes are not made in thinking around the progression and ongoing improvement of health care delivery for a continually changing society.

System modifications imposed from above can be a failure because they have not been thought about in sufficient detail, they were poorly researched. An example of this, I believe, was offering the GP's the option to drop out of hours care. From a management, strategic, view it probably saved money because it reduced the excess hours payment to doctors, who are expensive. But it has ended in the cumbersome and clinically inefficient out of hours NHS 111 telephone service, which in turn has provoked the appalling overuse of and delays in A & E departments. For the GP's it must have seemed an irresistible offer, but I think it has diminished and damaged their role within the society in their care.

Another example of a top-down change which, I think, was poorly managed was the introduction of electronic patient records, EPR, as a prelude to the so called "paperless hospital". Everyone, even an "IT Luddite" like myself, could see some advantage in patient notes and records being quickly available to all with the right of access, wherever they were, rather than being filed in a vast repository. The cost of withdrawing them and physically transporting them to wherever they were required, each time they were required, was enormous and the whole system was inefficient and unreliable. It was a perfect opportunity for a collaborative project with the commercial sector, introducing change in a researched and evolutionary fashion. Instead, groups of managers and clinicians with an interest in management were created, had a superficial look at various options and signed binding contracts with companies that really had no insight into clinical needs. The result was a prolonged period of frustration and dangerous confusion with a difficult to use and very difficult to modify system. Only by refusing to accept paper requests for investigations could all the clinicians be forced into using it.

Well designed and validated research is beginning to show that artificial intelligence, AI, can be more accurate and reliable in interpretation of clinical data than experienced clinicians in some specific fields, like imaging with MRI or CT scans. All very exciting, especially as the NHS is perfectly placed for this type of collaboration with industry.

It is human nature to be, to some extent, resistant to change unless it is quickly and obviously of benefit in some way. The pandemic has proved something that should have been obvious many years ago; there is a useful place for the telephone as a means of clinical follow-up for patients (but not for it to be the only doctor patient contact). Previously it was discouraged because the purchasing trust would not recognize it as a "clinical episode" and so the provider trust would not be paid for it. Madness!

It is my personal belief that the NHS, unless it undergoes some radical changes in structure, management and funding, will collapse in the not very distant future. If you have read my thoughts this far, without throwing the book away in disgust, you may agree that that would be a desperate loss to our society, in many ways. I have suggested several changes and I believe that they, or something like them, need to be implemented soon. But any change will have the best chance of being a success if the clinicians believe that it will bring real and lasting benefit to patients and, perhaps to a lesser extent, themselves. There is a psychological imperative to present changes in that way, which should be obvious, but not much attention seems to have been paid to that in the past. Top-down imposed changes will be justified by phrases like "improved efficiency", "greater control", "economic benefits", "resource management". But what the patients and most clinicians want to hear about are things like "greater safety", "better regulation", "simplicity of access", "reliable compliance" or "flexible staffing and delegation".

They may just be different ways of describing the same thing, most of the changes I have proposed are primarily no more than a change of habits and expectations, but some, obviously, will need to be implemented through political intervention. The single most important being the incorporation of all health care delivery, from conception to grave including social care, within the over-arching control of the NHS. The final completion of The National Health Service Act of 1946.

That is not a small undertaking, but if it can be seen to be in the public interest it would be widely accepted. As I have suggested, it would probably involve fewer compulsory purchase orders and less social disruption than building HS2 or a third runway at Heathrow/new London airport. Maybe those things will not be useful anyway post-covid.

The politicians must accept the need to put an end to the disruption of political interference from whatever Government happened to find itself in, always transient, power; in some way the NHS must be made largely self-governing and self-determining.

We need a national No Fault Compensation System. The politicians may not like this as so many of them have some legal background, but we need to bypass expensive lawyers who use patient sorrow or disappointment to generate a quagmire of anger, self-pity and bitterness, which usually turns out to be a frustratingly drawn out and unpleasant experience for everyone involved, except, perhaps, the lawyers. Anyone who has been truly damaged would be compensated appropriately by the NHS, under public scrutiny. Any clinician who was apparently undertaking dubious or illegal activities would be referred to the GMC or appropriate regulatory authority.

Abolish the private, profiteering, staffing agencies (a type of modern slavery). They will be replaced by well-regulated NHS Trust Staff Banks.

Abolish private health insurance schemes, financial scams for profit which, in terms of genuine "health care" do much harm for no benefit, except to the financiers. They are totally unnecessary in the UK, let the rest of the world swill in its own health care cesspool.

The other changes are no more than cultural ones in professional behaviour from the various groups of NHS staff or the expectations of society generally.

All clinical work, both public and private, would be undertaken within the NHS, with greater probity in private practice, together with more transparent and reputable regulation. This, in turn, would bring additional income to the state system, perhaps to help improve the working environment for staff. It would also give the managers better metrics for assessing good and bad performance, enabling them to employ the incentive of the carrot, not just the deterrent of the stick. It is difficult, at present to quantify bad performance, so it is usually ignored.

Abandon the pretense that nursing is primarily an academic career, requiring a university degree on enrollment. Make being a student nurse more interesting, more inclusive within the life of the principal training hospital. They would make a productive contribution to the clinical workload, for which they should be paid enough to have a reasonable quality of life whilst studying.

Abandon the relatively recent practice of rating the ability to pass exams as the sole criterion for a place at medical school. Other aspects of endeavour and ability should also be considered, as was formerly the case. Identify those junior doctors who show a penchant for management, then start training them early in the appropriate skills, making NHS management a serious clinical speciality.

It seems to me that it is vital to re-engage and enthuse the GPs. They have lost their essential core role of being the first point of contact for everyone in their community with a non- acutely traumatic clinical concern. To some extent the politicians stripped that from them, but I think they should, somehow, be persuaded to take back an out of hours on-call commitment. There are too few of them, but that problem must be exacerbated by the fact that so many of them only want to work part time or retire young. Some practices are always able to offer prompt appointments on request, I do not really know why others cannot. There is, of course, a huge range of demographic variations; but that is a problem the NHS will always have to cope with.

I do know that one source of profound frustration for the GPs is their difficulty interacting with the specialists of their local hospitals. This is, at least in part, the consequence of the politicians trying to hide waiting times for specialist referrals with their absurd "choose and book" system. The GPs should revert to being the gatekeepers for specialist referrals, a task they used to perform extremely well. Professional relationships between the GPs and their local specialist hospital colleagues must be rebuilt.

Hospital food should be pleasant and nutritious, for the patients and the staff. Why not encourage families and friends to contribute to a patient's hospital care by arranging their meals, under the distant supervision of the ward nurses? Encouraging family involvement in care has many benefits.

Why should the staff not have the privacy to eat something during a break, without having to compete with visitors to purchase it, in a long queue?

The population of The UK must learn to stop regarding The NHS as the pinnacle comfort zone of The

Nanny State, something they have a right to access in any circumstances and to complain about at will and with impunity. It would be a start if they began to appreciate that a nanny state is really a totalitarian dictatorship wolf in the sheep's clothing of a caring society. Back to Orwell and Big Brother, "freedom is not being able to do what you want to, it is wanting to do what you are allowed to". A very cynical and dangerous premise.

It is a simple truth that in "western, first world cultures" people value, above many things, something that they feel they have paid for; a sense of ownership, which entails a feeling of caring and responsibility. Give people the option to pay, not extortionately, but proportionately, for their treatment; they would be far more grateful and appreciative, as well as it being an extra income stream.

Before the beginning of 2020 I had no doubt that, although the people of the UK were glad for the existence of the NHS, society at large had no real insight into the difficulties the NHS was facing or the worsening struggle of the clinicians to maintain services. Morale was low and sinking fast and there was no sign of the management doing anything that was not to their own advantage, or politicians having any ideas beyond vying with each other as to who would throw the most money into the black hole.

The people did not appreciate or really value the NHS and they had very unrealistic ideas of what a State Health Care Delivery System should offer.

One of the observations that has most annoyed me over the last 40 years (made by occasional patients and, sadly, sometimes by non-medical friends) is "so and so has been rather let down by the NHS". Inevitably I know of cases where patients have been "let down" by individual clinicians but none where somebody has been "let down" by the NHS. The reality is that society, of which the NHS should be an exemplary part, has "let down" the NHS. It has been badly financed (which is not the same as being underfunded), badly structured and saddest of all, badly abused by the community which it has struggled to serve.

Public funding post-pandemic will be tighter than ever. Health care funding must be re-structured with innovative sources of funding and those that profit in a non-contributary way should be eliminated.

The Coronavirus Pandemic seems to have made the public genuinely appreciate the work and commitment of the health care frontline. But the Panic of The Pandemic has had health care consequences that will stretch far beyond the complex struggle to control infection rates and minimize morbidity and mortality. Basic clinical care was crushed beneath the spinning wheels of under-staffing, unremitting stress for the front-line and constant fear of viral transmission. People were afraid to seek medical advice and so diagnoses were missed. The health care delivery systems were literally petrified to perform their routine activities by fear of emergency admissions, so treatments were postponed or abandoned.

It was a situation where it is human nature to fall back on routines, habits and responses that have been ingrained by practice, experience and training. An emergency that above all calls for teamwork; like the creation, purchase, production and distribution of a vaccine.

This is the exact opposite of the distrust of teams and the ethos of protocols and bureaucracy imposed on the clinicians over many years by NHS management. Not only are protocols dangerous because they discourage clinicians from thinking on an individual case basis, but they also create a hazard if there are just too many of them. A surfeit of protocols to follow, forms to complete and boxes to tick will inevitably result in the people charged with the task becoming indifferent to them. In the end it is difficult to think of any form as an important piece of clinical documentation, particularly in an unusually stressful situation.

An example of an important document is the DNACPR form. This stands for Do Not Attempt Cardio-Pulmonary Resuscitation, it is a heavy and very blunt clinical tool and like all such tools it can be both useful and dangerous. It is intended to prevent wasted or unwanted (by the patient) time and energy being expended trying to prolong the life of a patient where it has a negligible chance of success or, if successful, could not result in a meaningful prolongation of life in a form that would be acceptable to the patient, either in the patient's own opinion or (if the patient cannot express an opinion) in the judgement of their next of kin or the holder of a power of attorney.

It is quite short for a document with such irrevocable consequences, but its complexities may be considerable. It is important to complete it thoughtfully, not as a box-ticking exercise and it should be completed or counter-signed by the consultant in clinical charge.

A 64-year-old woman is admitted as an emergency, by ambulance from her home, with drowsiness and mild confusion. She was dispatched into the ambulance by her husband and daughter who are, of course, not allowed to accompany her. On testing, the ambulance crew had found that she had low oxygen levels and there is a clear history of contact with someone who had subsequently tested positive for covid 19.

On arrival in hospital the diagnosis of covid pneumonia is confirmed. She is admitted direct to a respiratory high dependency unit (HDU) and pressurized oxygen is prescribed and administered. An HDU is one step down from an Intensive Therapy Unit (ITU), which is usually reserved for ventilation under anaesthesia. The consultant respiratory physician calls the husband at home, to update him and promises to call early the next morning, which she does.

This is exemplary clinical management and communication; just as was rendered unto The Prime Minister himself.

The woman spends 8 nights on the respiratory HDU, which is tough, but she is medicated and nursed through it and is transferred to a routine covid isolation ward, where she is still allowed no visitors. But her family have been able to speak with her every day, as well as to nursing and medical staff. If requested the nurses would even arrange a video link.

After about another week in isolation she is considered to no longer be an infection risk and she is transferred to a standard medical ward where she can have a visitor for one hour a day by appointment. Most of the other patients in the ward are, like her, post-covid. After about another week she is well enough to be discharged home, with appropriate follow-up arranged and her family are allowed to collect her.

She is supplied with some medication to take home and an envelope containing relevant instructions and a copy of her discharge summary, as sent to her GP. Her family are very relieved to get her home as they have been well aware that she has co-morbidities that clearly place her in a high-risk category for a fatal outcome from covid infection. She has a rare progressive neurological condition called spino-cerebellar-ataxia. This is similar in effect to, but less aggressive than, the more widely known condition of motor neurone disease and is not, in itself, necessarily fatal. She is wheelchair dependent with some speech impairment and has become moderately obese. She also has known pelvic secondaries from a uterine cancer resected 6 years earlier. These are slow growing but not amenable to any form of curative treatment.

They are therefore not surprised, when going through her discharge papers, to find a completed DNACPR form, any clinician should know that her chance of surviving mechanical ventilation (being transferred to an ITU) are zero. In fact, her husband had specifically requested that she should not be transferred to ITU; his exact words were, to several of the doctors involved in her care, "HDU is good. ITU is the road to hell". They had all agreed and it is very sensible, from the hospital's point of view and for continuity of care, to complete a DNACPR form. But the family are astonished by *the specific statements and instructions made in completing the form. The patient herself has no recollection of being asked about the form, which is not surprising; the form is dated for the evening of her admission.*

I need to go through the form to explain their surprise, but I need only cover some of it.

There are 4 sections requiring some responses and this is done on the Electronic Patient Records, EPR.

1.Reason for DNACPR decision.

There are 3 choices, A, B and C; A or B would have been appropriate in this case and A was selected. CPR is unlikely to be successful due to: METASTATIC OVARIAN CANCER WITH LIFE EXPECTANCY OF 1 TO 2 YEARS. POOR FUNCTIONAL BASELINE.

LILAC FORM STAYS WITH PERSON WHEREVER THEY ARE BEING CARED FOR. WHITE FORMS FOR AUDIT AND NOTES.

UNIFIED DO NOT ATTEMPT CARDIOPULMONARY RESUSCITATION (DNACPR)

In the event of cardiac or respiratory arrest no attempts at CPR will be made. All other appropriate treatment and care will be provided.

Name: ▮▮▮	Date of DNACPR Decision ▮▮▮	**NHS** South of England
Address: ▮▮▮	www.southofengland.nhs.uk/what we are doing/end of life care	
D.O.B: ▮▮▮	**Institution Name** Form completed electronically? Yes ☒ No ☐	
NHS or Hospital No: ▮▮▮	Before completing this form, please see explanation notes.	

1. Reason for DNACPR decision

☒ A) CPR is unlikely to be successful due to: Metastatic ovarian cancer with life expectancy of 1 to 2 years. Poor functional baseline.

The person has been informed of the decision: Yes ☒   No ☐   If No state reason:

The relevant other has been informed of the decision: Yes ☐   No ☒   If No state reason: Other: n/a

Name of relevant other: unknown

☐ B) CPR maybe successful, but followed by a length and quality of life which would not be of overall benefit to the person.

• Person involved in discussions?   Yes ☐   No ☐   If No state reason:

• Person lacks mental capacity and has a legally appointed Welfare Attorney: Name:

• Person lacks mental capacity and does not have a legally appointed Welfare Attorney. Decision is made on the balance of overall benefit to the person in discussion with: Name(s):

☐ C) There is a valid advance decision to refuse CPR in the following circumstances: All circumstances   Yes ☐   No ☐

Specific Circumstances (please state):

Attach a copy of the Advance Decision to Refuse Treatment (ADRT) to the back of the DNACPR form.

This is correct and appropriate, except that pelvic secondaries are unlikely to affect cardio-pulmonary function.

The person has been informed of the decision: Yes / No, YES SELECTED.

Again, not inappropriate, except that the person was confused leaving home and is likely to be more confused after admission to a hospital, so may not be able to give informed consent. Indeed, she was not.

The relevant other has been informed of the decision: Yes / No, NO SELECTED. If No state reason: OTHER: N/A. Name of relevant other: UNKNOWN.

Possibly true as the form was being completed, but only because of not looking in EPR where it is clearly recorded. Given the probable physical and emotional state of the person at the time, I feel this is a particularly silly error, but to do things correctly would have taken some time in a highly time-pressurised environment.

2.Healthcare professional making this DNACPR decision.

This section was completed, electronically by a trainee doctor.

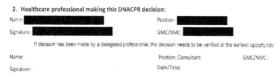

The form was completed by a "delegated professional".

However frenetic and fraught the first few days were, the person was an inpatient for over 3 weeks and consultant ward rounds occur at least once every working day.

The form was never "verified" by a "Consultant".

This is another golf ball flying through a tree; here is the first potential opportunity to correct an initially fairly harmless mistake.

3. Review: (Select ONE box only): This is an indefinite decision / Needs reviewing, INDEFINITE DECISION SELECTED.

3. Review: (Select ONE box only)	☒ This is an indefinite decision	☐ Needs reviewing
Review date:	Outcome of review: DNACPR to continue? Yes ☐ No ☐	
Name:	Position:	
Signature:		

4. Who has been informed of this DNACPR decision?

4. Who has been informed of this DNACPR decision?		
☐ GP	☐ Ambulance Warning Flag	☐ Out of Hours
☒ Care Provider (Please state):		
Other (Please state):	Other: none	

The only thing marked is the "Care Provider", but it is not stated who that is considered to be. The completion of the form has not been discussed with the GP or, more importantly, the family, who are declared by the way in which the form has been completed, to be "unknown, not applicable or non-existent". They have "been informed", but only by the fact that the form has been sent to them, amongst other documents.

The golf ball has flown through the tree and the last two sections have been completed in a way that could allow it to land in a very unpleasant bunker.

This is my last clinical scenario; it is the only one that I can categorically state is factually correct as described. I can do this because there is no risk of my breaching patient confidentiality; the patient is my wife, I am her "unknown" relevant other.

We feel nothing but overwhelming admiration, sympathy and above all gratitude for all the front-line people involved in my wife's care; from the telephonist taking the first call and the ambulance crew, through all the doctors and nurses, to the pharmacist and therapists who supported her discharge home. We have no quibble with the junior doctor who completed the DNACPR form, it was appropriate at the time of admission. But it is lodged in a patient's electronic clinical record and is impossible to remove; it is a criminal offence to erase or alter clinical notes retrospectively. It can be counter-manded, but, as we have seen, people do not always have the time to peruse the records carefully in a clinical emergency.

My wife is, fortunately, in no danger. She has sufficient family and friends to ensure that if she were admitted to hospital for some other emergency there would be no misunderstanding. That is not always the case.

No one knows how long they may live, the question that the DNACPR form is intended to address is whether they wish to continue living, as they are or may become. Many people who ask, or are offered the choice, to complete that form are not in a happy social environment that includes family and friends. But even if knowingly and willingly completed by a patient the question of what constitutes "informed consent" must be considered, just as with a consent to treatment form. Anybody with no insight into health care delivery cannot truly give informed consent in a way that can be captured by any form or protocol. Informed consent is an agreement, an understanding between the patient or their advocate and the clinician responsible for their care and wellbeing.

When my wife was admitted with covid infection she and all her loved ones agreed that, if it was to be her fate to die from it, there should be no "heroic" attempts to prolong her life; no consignment to mechanical ventilation on an ITU. But if her destiny were to survive it and she was to return to her own home, where she is very much the centre of family life, where she lives, with some support from her family but no outside support services, a fully intellectually and emotionally independent life then, although she may not have long to live, she has a lot to live for in whatever time remains to her.

That cannot really be summarised in a one size fits all form, because of the infinite variety of human beliefs, aspirations and circumstances. So, the form, the heavy, blunt, useful and dangerous instrument, can only be a signpost. Any actual decision about a patient's clinical management must be based on trust and understanding. During my wife's admission with covid pneumonia we felt that trust and understanding and will always be grateful for it. The potential misunderstanding that could have arisen from the detail of the form's completion was the result of the understaffed and overworked clinicians being so engulfed in silly forms that they had not the energy to pay attention to the one important one. There was no diminution of actual clinical care and, of course, no management review of whether the form had been appropriately completed. We will not be asking for such a review to be conducted, it would only result in another layer of bureaucracy.

The NHS has become, over the last 20 years or more, an increasingly stressful and difficult environment in which to work. There are many contributory reasons for this, not least perhaps, that the world in general has become more complex and stressful, but a major reason is that NHS management have become obsessed with bureaucratic forms and rigid protocols. Life as a clinician in health care is naturally stressful, most worthwhile jobs are to a greater or lesser degree, but the intrinsic stress is multiplied enormously by the endless, overwhelming bureaucracy, the need to fill in forms and the knowledge that if they are not filled in (it does not matter if they are filled in correctly or not) there will be unpleasant consequences.

If a flawed and innately unnecessarily stressful pattern of work is applied to any endeavour an extraneous increase in stress levels is likely to tip it into failure, sometimes catastrophically. In my opinion the NHS was approaching the point of collapse long before the pandemic, but it will have been severely damaged by its consequences. It will take some years for the extent of the damage to be realized, let alone repaired, but perhaps the pandemic could precipitate some much-needed reforms.

Indeed, the pandemic will probably change the manner in which we live forever. It could have as big an effect as the development of the wheel or the invention of the printing press. Future historians may reflect on The Pandemic Revolution in the same way that we consider The Agricultural, The Industrial or The Technological Revolutions.

If we are lucky and our Leaders are wise it could be a change for enormous good; a more caring, less selfish and destructive society, an abhorrence of crime, restoration of family values – perhaps the great question of April and May 2020, "why are so many people in Care Homes dying?" goes a word too far and should just be "why are so many people in Care Homes?".

If we have learnt nothing people will quickly forget their gratitude to our health care delivery systems; already there is growing dissatisfaction with the non-Covid performance of the NHS during the pandemic. That risks a huge rebound of disappointment and despair amongst the frontline workforce, who have already suffered so much. They may well leave and if they do Eden will have burnt.

The present situation represents a great opportunity to end Eden's struggle with the firewall forever. We have a Prime Minister who, perhaps, is capable of thinking outside the box and he has a large enough majority (I do not really care what Party he leads) to avoid the frustrations of obstructionist Party Politics. But, the nature of politics being what it is, by the time of (or shortly after) going to press that Government may already have fallen. The public, in the warm glow of gratitude to the NHS, may be in a receptive mood to accept the limitations of what could be free at the time of need. Or, that gratitude may have already reverted to the previous resentful perceived grievances. However, they may still be realizing that a well-run NHS will always be preferable to any form of private health care delivery. The NHS clinicians were perfectly positioned to deal with a pandemic, but it is now clear that they were hopelessly under-powered and poorly managed.

No single individual will identify all the possible answers to all the difficulties of an all-embracing health care system, certainly not me, but I hope I have identified some weaknesses and anomalies within the present structure and outlined some plausible solutions.

I wonder if anything will change.

Why not sign up to our mailing list here:

Why not browse our BOOKSHOP?

More about Bite-Sized Books here:

Printed in Great Britain
by Amazon

82706833R00132